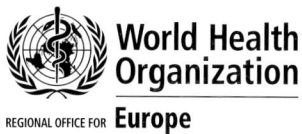

Addressing the social determinants of health:
the urban dimension and the role of local government

Abstract

This report summarizes the evidence on the social determinants of health and the built environment with special reference to the role of local government across countries in the WHO European Region. It draws on the findings of the global Commission on Social Determinants of Health and the European review of social determinants of health and the health divide. Through its leadership, local government has a significant role to play in working across sectors and with civil society partners to support and accelerate action to address the social determinants of health and the causes of health inequalities. The evidence presented here provides the background to the complementary report *Healthy cities tackle the social determinants of inequities in health: a framework for action*.

Keywords

URBAN HEALTH
LOCAL GOVERNMENT
SOCIOECONOMIC FACTORS
HEALTHCARE DISPARITIES
PATIENT ADVOCACY
EUROPE

Address requests about publications of the WHO Regional Office for Europe to:
  Publications
  WHO Regional Office for Europe
  Scherfigsvej 8
  DK-2100 Copenhagen Ø, Denmark
Alternatively, complete an online request form for documentation, health information, or for permission to quote or translate, on the Regional Office web site (http://www.euro.who.int/pubrequest).

ISBN 978 92 890 0269 1

© World Health Organization 2012

All rights reserved. The Regional Office for Europe of the World Health Organization welcomes requests for permission to reproduce or translate its publications, in part or in full.

The designations employed and the presentation of the material in this publication do not imply the expression of any opinion whatsoever on the part of the World Health Organization concerning the legal status of any country, territory, city or area or of its authorities, or concerning the delimitation of its frontiers or boundaries. Dotted lines on maps represent approximate border lines for which there may not yet be full agreement.

The mention of specific companies or of certain manufacturers' products does not imply that they are endorsed or recommended by the World Health Organization in preference to others of a similar nature that are not mentioned. Errors and omissions excepted, the names of proprietary products are distinguished by initial capital letters.

All reasonable precautions have been taken by the World Health Organization to verify the information contained in this publication. However, the published material is being distributed without warranty of any kind, either express or implied. The responsibility for the interpretation and use of the material lies with the reader. In no event shall the World Health Organization be liable for damages arising from its use. The views expressed by authors, editors, or expert groups do not necessarily represent the decisions or the stated policy of the World Health Organization.

Edited by Mike Grady and Peter Goldblatt,
Institute of Health Equity, University College London,
United Kingdom

Text editing: David Breuer
Book design: Sven Lund
Cover design: Christophe Lanoux, Paris, France

Cover photos: Monkey Business Images/Dreamstime.com; Poznyakov/Dreamstime.com: Jon Furniss; michaeljung/Fotolia.com; Lupoalb68/Dreamstime.com; keribevan/Fotolia.com

Contents

Foreword v

1. Introduction 1

2. How the report of the Commission on Social Determinants of Health and the strategic review of health inequalities in England post-2010 apply to urban settings 9

3. Local government and the social determinants of health: an overview of policy and practice in the European Region 21

4. Final conclusions and implications for the WHO European Healthy Cities Network 39

References 45

Foreword

The scientific evidence on the social determinants of health is complex and multifaceted. It is addressed to a wide range of stakeholders within and beyond the health sector and all levels of government. This report focuses on the social determinants of health in the urban context and explores the role of local government in nurturing psychosocial well-being and resilience at both the individual and population levels. It draws on the findings of several key studies at the global and European Region levels and provides a helpful overview of practices from across Europe. The report covers priority action areas and identifies key implementation issues of particular relevance to creating healthy and sustainable places and communities. Increasing evidence shows that local governments and civil society are increasingly interested in being sensitive and proactive in tackling inequities. Further, there is high demand for publications that are tailored to the urban and local perspectives. I am convinced this well-written publication will make a difference to all those who are interested in these perspectives.

I would like to express my deep appreciation to Mike Grady and Peter Goldblatt, University College London, United Kingdom, who edited this publication on behalf of the WHO Regional Office for Europe. Many thanks to all the colleagues who contributed in the writing, including Hugh Barton, Caroline Bird and Marcus Grant, WHO Collaborating Centre for Healthy Urban Environments, University of the West of England, Bristol, United Kingdom; Ruth Bell, Institute of Health Equity, University College London, United Kingdom; Jeni Bremner, Paul Giepmans and Elisabeth Jelfs, European Health Management Association, Brussels, Belgium; Liam Hughes, Local Government Association, London, United Kingdom; and Di McNeish, DMSS Research & Consultancy, Whitchurch, United Kingdom. Special thanks are also due to all the members of the WHO European Healthy Cities Network and European national healthy cities networks, which provided helpful feedback throughout the drafting process.

Agis D. Tsouros

Head, Policy and Cross-Cutting Programmes and Regional Director's Special Projects
WHO Regional Office for Europe

1. Introduction

1.1 Global and European Union context

The publication of the report of the WHO Commission on Social Determinants of Health in 2008 *(1)* represented a key milestone in the increasing international attention paid to the fundamental importance of social determinants for health status. As the report concludes *(1)*: "Action is needed on the determinants of health – from structural conditions of society to the daily conditions in which people grow, live and work at all levels from global to local, across government and inclusive of all stakeholders from civil society and the private sector." The importance of addressing the social determinants of health and health inequities[1] has also found increasing attention within European Union (EU) policy-making. In part, the implicit importance of improving the social determinants of health has been anchored in the Lisbon Strategy for Growth and Jobs through its commitment to productivity, employment and education, but the social determinants of health and their importance in tackling inequalities in health have also been explicitly highlighted at the EU level, most recently by the incoming Commissioner for Health and Consumer Affairs, John Dalli, in his pre-inauguration hearings before the European Parliament in January 2010 *(3)*. Inequalities in health in general have also received significantly greater policy attention at the EU level in recent years. Tackling inequalities in health is one of the key priorities of the European Commission's health strategy, *Together for health: a strategic approach for the EU 2008–2013 (4)*. The publication of a European Commission communication on solidarity in health and reducing health inequalities in the EU in October 2009 *(5)* is therefore a significant step forward in pushing forward EU action on inequalities in health.

This report explores the priority issues, the evidence base and future policy direction needed to address the social determinants of health in the urban context, with particular reference to the role of local government. Chapter 2 sets out evidence on the social determinants of health and the built environment and Chapter 3 provides examples of local government activity across the social gradient from several countries in the WHO European Region. It provides the background to *Healthy cities tackle the social determinants of inequities in health: a framework for action (6)* for the members of the Network of European Healthy Cities Networks and the members of the WHO European Healthy Cities Network, which are committed to delivering the overarching goal of Phase V (2009–2013) of health and health equity in all local policies.

This report and the framework for action *(6)* were formally presented in three seminars at the 2010 Annual Integrated Business and Technical Conference of the WHO European Healthy Cities Network and the Network of European Healthy Cities Networks in Sandnes, Norway in June 2010 as part of a wide consultation process.

---

[1] The report of the Commission on Social Determinants of Health *(1)* defined health inequities as systematic differences in health considered to be avoidable by reasonable action and therefore unfair, in accordance with the WHO definition of health inequities *(2)* as "avoidable inequalities in health between groups of people within countries and between countries". Various actors in this field prefer to use health inequality (and inequalities) and others health inequity (and inequities) to refer to these avoidable differences in health. These actors mostly agree on using the word equity as the positive term (health equity, equity in health) and not equality.

This report also links with and will feed into the European review of the social determinants of health and the health divide commissioned by the WHO Regional Office for Europe in 2010, which produced a consultation report in June 2011 and is producing a final report and recommendations in 2012.

1.2 Context in the European Region

The WHO European Region has 53 Member States with almost 900 million people living in a wide variety of social, economic, political and cultural contexts. There are a variety of regional and county structures and thousands of municipalities. Although the Region has the highest average score on the Human Development Index of any WHO region, significant inequities in health remain within and between countries and population groups *(7)*.

The European health report 2009 (7) shows that health status indicators such as mortality continue to improve across Europe, but there are still dramatic differences in health between subregions and groups within countries, closely linked to degrees of social disadvantage.[2]

The European Region is also going through a period of great change and uncertainty, especially because of the global economic downturn. With economic growth unlikely to recover soon, debt will constrain public finances across the European Region for many years and may adversely affect local government funding. The consequent unemployment and public spending cuts will affect the living conditions of millions of people in the European Region and will have the greatest impact on the most disadvantaged people. Unless action is taken, recession may wipe out recent progress and further increase inequities in health. The role of local government becomes even more important, especially in cities and urban areas, with a vital role to play in fostering and enhancing local health, well-being and resilience.

1.3 WHO European Healthy Cities Network and national healthy cities networks

WHO launched Healthy Cities in 1987 in the European Region as a vehicle to bring the strategy for Health for All to the local level of government. From its beginning, the Healthy Cities project recognized that health is determined by a range of personal, social, economic and environmental factors. Today it is a global public health movement at the local level, and within the WHO European Region, almost 100 cities are members of the WHO European Healthy Cities Network, and more than 1500 cities are members of national networks in 30 countries in the European Region.

The Healthy Cities project has evolved over more than two decades in response to new urban health challenges, and at its core is a coherent set of enduring qualities, elements and goals. Healthy cities give explicit political commitment to improving their citizens' health. They acknowledge major health challenges and the economic, physical and social factors that influence them. Cities participating in the WHO European Healthy Cities Network actively explore ways of implementing strategies at the local level to address the wider social determinants of health from which inequities in health arise. Local governments provide essential public health leadership and are committed to creating the preconditions for healthier living and participatory governance and to facilitating intersectoral action to achieve greater health and equity in health.

The overarching theme for Phase V (2009–2013) is health and health equity in all local policies. Health in all policies recognizes that population health is not merely a product of health sector programmes but largely determined by policies and actions beyond the

---

[2] Examples of widening gaps reported in *The European health report 2009 (7)* include the spread of multidrug-resistant tuberculosis and environmental health problems due to air pollution in urban industrial centres and the combustion of solid fuel in homes.

health sector. Health in all policies addresses policies such as those influencing transport, housing and urban development, the environment, education, agriculture, finance, taxation and economic development. In implementing health and health equity in all local policies, Phase V builds on previous city health development planning and draws on the conclusions and recommendations of the global Commission on Social Determinants of Health *(1)*.

1.4 Role of local government in tackling the social determinants of health

Within these overarching developments, the particular role of local government in tackling the social determinants of health and equity in health has been increasingly recognized. In particular, at the EU level it has been acknowledged that local government can make a vital contribution by fostering exchange of good practice and measuring progress *(4)*. Other international actors (WHO and the Commission on Social Determinants of Health *(8)*) have also highlighted the importance of action taken by local government and the interplay between local and national government in tackling the social determinants of health.

Two key reasons underpin this recognition.

First, the social model of health is being given increased attention; it emphasizes good health results from positive socioeconomic and environmental factors, with health largely being socially determined *(9)*. In contrast to the curative, medical model of health, many of whose determinants lie within the purview of the health care sector (which may or may not be controlled by local government), local government usually has primary responsibility for planning and/or delivering many of the services that are crucial to addressing the social determinants of health: education, transport, housing and urban planning. The literature highlights the fact that local authorities are also often in a strong position to bring a wide variety of local actors around the table to stimulate action in a way that the health care sector alone cannot *(10)*. The framework for action *(6)* outlines action to develop collaborative working between local authorities and partners (framework for action: sections 4.3, 5.2, 5.4, 5.7.4, 5.8.2 and 6.1).

Second, some commentators argue that the structures underpinning local government, especially decentralization, have inherent potential to stimulate change by reducing central influence and promoting local autonomy. As Litvack et al. *(11)* have shown, reducing central influences and promoting local autonomy may lead to more flexible and efficient policies, as local authorities are better able to respond to local needs and may have greater knowledge of and sensitivity to local problems. As de Vries *(12)* has argued, centralized systems are tempted to impose decisional overload as decision-makers try to overrule the complexity of local problems.

Local authorities can play an important role in making decisions and implementing policy on the social determinants of health and have the potential to be key actors in reducing inequities in health and improving social welfare for citizens in the European Region. However, local government also faces several challenges in taking practical action on improving the social determinants of health and tackling inequities in health.

- Although local government may be better placed to respond to local needs, it is always situated within a wider legislative context that creates the conditions that shape its ability to act.
- Localization, decentralization and delegated powers may bring tension between different levels of government (vertical conflicts) or between different local government agencies (horizontal conflicts). Problems in securing the alignment of overall national policy objectives with subnational interventions and local project objectives may undermine coherence and synergy.
- It cannot necessarily be assumed that local govern-

ment has sufficient capacity and resources to maximize health gain through the social determinants of health and to carry out policies for the social determinants for which they are responsible *(10,12)*.

Chapter 3 explores these issues, including examples of action by local government, in interviews with key stakeholders.

1.5 Which social determinants of health are especially linked to urban or city settings?

Healthy cities tackle the social determinants of inequities in health: a framework for action (6) sets out the role of city authorities in addressing the social determinants of health and equity in health through the medium of people, process and place (Fig. 1). It points out that, in cities, authorities are responsible for a particular place and for the health and well-being of the residents, migrants and visitors. The city authorities also have varying degrees of responsibility or potential to affect many of the processes occurring within that place (administrative, regulative, planning, commercial and social processes).

Fig. 1. Addressing the social determinants of health through place, process and people

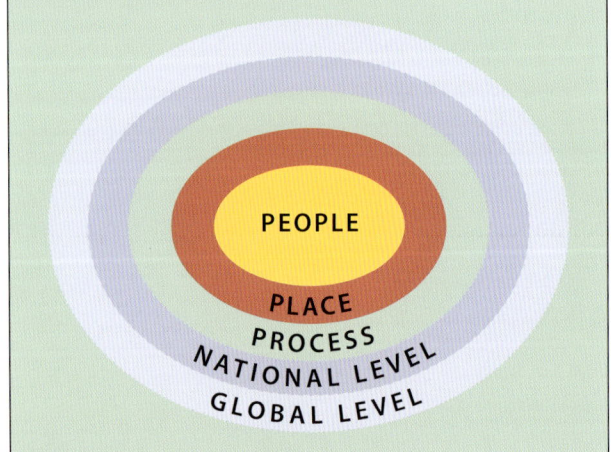

Source: *Healthy cities tackle the social determinants of inequities in health: a framework for action (6)*.

The built and natural environment is an important determinant of health. This applies especially to population groups disadvantaged by relative poverty, unemployment, low status, gender, sexual orientation, ethnicity or disability. They typically have fewer choices open to them and are in locations and settings that are less conducive to good health, with little ability to move away from unhealthy working and living environments. The evidence *(1)* shows a social gradient in the population groups living in areas with the least favourable environmental conditions and the need for investment in new and existing housing across the social gradient. Studies in the early 2000s *(13)* used the term environmental justice to describe spatial patterns in which disadvantage and poor environmental quality coincide. Several reviews *(14)* indicate that people with low income are more likely to live in poor-quality built environments (including increased exposure to health risks from noise and poor air quality), and this contributes to poor health. Layers of health risk can also overlap. Children and older people are especially vulnerable not only because of biological vulnerability but also because of the significant numbers of children and older people who have low income.

However, spatial variation can be associated with a huge divergence in health outcomes. Key spatial mechanisms that affect this include transport; air pollution; road safety; neighbourhoods and facilities; housing and urban planning; green space; crime and the fear of crime; and the urban environment and climate.

1.5.1 Transport

Families with lower income tend to have lower mobility but greater exposure to the adverse environmental conditions related to transport such as air and noise pollution and road traffic. People who are more deprived are also more susceptible to these harmful health effects because of greater vulnerability to illness associated with the other social determinants of health. Access to transport that enables residents to move outside of their own community has been shown to positively correlate with a reduced fear of social isolation and positive mental health *(15)*.

1.5.2 Air pollution

Air pollution most severely affects disadvantaged people, with increased risk of respiratory diseases and other illness. Greater air pollution has been linked to deprived neighbourhoods in several countries, including Norway *(16)*. Other studies have highlighted that even cities that might not follow this trend where people with higher socioeconomic status are exposed to the highest pollution concentrations, mortality rates from air pollution–related causes are still highest among those with lower socioeconomic status, indicating greater susceptibility to the effects of air pollution among the most deprived people *(17)*.

1.5.3 Road safety

Globally, road crashes are the single largest cause of unintentional injury, despite preventive strategies being in place *(8)*. Death and serious injury from road crashes vary greatly by socioeconomic status. A study in England *(18)* showed that children in the most deprived 10% of areas are four times more likely to be hit by a car as children in the least deprived 10%. Children aged 0–19 years and people older than 60 years are especially vulnerable to injury through road crashes.

1.5.4 Neighbourhoods and facilities

Urban land-use patterns are one of the main influences on the levels of physical activity, especially among lower-income groups who get much of their physical activity through daily living activity and travel rather than recreation *(19)*. Access to local facilities such as shops, schools, health centres and places of informal recreation are important for health and well-being, both for the physical activity taken in getting there and the social interaction on the way there or at the facilities. This is especially important for people who get much of their physical activity from walking rather than recreation. However, disadvantaged areas disproportionately experience the deteriorating features of an urban environment such as dilapidation, vandalism, graffiti and litter, leading to a sense of insecurity on streets and in parks and play areas. This means that people in these areas use these facilities less than elsewhere, and children are less likely to be let out to play. This leads to reduced physical activity and exacerbates health problems such as obesity. A secondary analysis of a cross-sectional survey of 12 cities in Europe *(20)* found that respondents from areas with high levels of litter and graffiti were 50% less likely than respondents from areas with low levels to be physically active and 50% more likely to be overweight.

1.5.5 Housing and urban planning

Households with lower income are more likely to occupy low-quality housing, which is more difficult and more expensive to heat, illustrating the spatial segregation of cities. Extra deaths between December and March are attributed to cold weather, with children, older people and people with long-term illnesses being the most vulnerable. Rising fuel prices exacerbate the problem for people in poorly insulated homes, causing more fuel poverty and worsening health. Environmental noise problems can also lead to sleep disturbance, cardiovascular disease and impaired mental health, and this is more severe in areas of deprivation and in the areas of high-density housing and other accommodation commonly occupied by people with lower income.

1.5.6 Green space

The available evidence *(21)* indicates the many benefits of green space for both physical and mental health and well-being. These include decreases in general health problems, blood pressure, cholesterol and stress levels and improved perceived general health and resilience.

Evidence *(21)* shows that inequality in mortality is lower in population groups living in the greenest areas. However, green space is not equally available to all the population, with neighbourhoods with low-income residents often lacking in green space or with poorly maintained, vandalized or unsafe green areas. The benefits of increases in physical activity and improved mental health only arise if the green spaces are of high quality, accessible and safe.

According to several reviews *(14)*, access to green spaces and nature positively affects mental health, possibly by reducing stress and by providing distraction and distancing people from their everyday activities. In addition, green spaces promote social interaction and cohesion. Conversely, restricted access to green spaces has been associated with poorer mental health. Residents in urban social housing who had views of trees and open spaces demonstrated a greater capacity to cope with stress than residents who did not have such access. Older people in particular benefit from such access. Access to green space also has an accentuated positive effect on physical health for people with low income *(22)*.

Incorporating accessible and safe green space into urban neighbourhood design increases use and positively influences levels of physical activity, mental well-being and resilience and the perceived risk of crime *(23)*.

1.5.7 Crime and the fear of crime

One of the main social effects related to urban form is residents' perceived fear of violence or crime *(24)*. This has been shown to negatively affect mental health. The groups who feel most vulnerable include women, especially mothers with low income and those with mental health problems *(14)*. Perceptions of safety are influenced by fear of street crime but also by injury from road traffic crashes and a reaction to the aesthetic impression, which includes the presence of graffiti, litter and state of disrepair of the surrounding community *(23)*. This disrepair is disproportionately high in low-income and disadvantaged areas *(14)*.

Evidence *(15)* shows that crime and the fear of crime can cause residents to experience time–space inequality. This has been shown to result in poor mental health, including feelings of social isolation, negative mood and low self-esteem.

Time–space inequality describes the variation in the ability of community residents to access and use spaces both within their immediate and wider environment at different times during the day or night. This was less prevalent among mentally healthy men or middle-income women. Time–space inequality seemed to be diminished by interventions that encourage spatial and temporal movements and encourage connectivity to a wider geography, such as comprehensive local public transport systems and government-issued free travel passes for vulnerable population groups.

1.5.8 The urban environment and climate

Healthy and sustainable cities have a shared policy agenda in mitigating climate change, although the impact of climate change will vary across the Region. Two specific aspects of climate change are likely to significantly affect the urban environment and disproportionately influence disadvantaged people, potentially increasing inequities in health and reducing social cohesion: increasing temperatures and flooding.

Exposure to heat causes illness and death in the urban environment. People with lower socioeconomic status and ethnic minority groups are more likely to live in warmer neighbourhoods and experience greater exposure to heat stress and drought. High settlement density, sparse vegetation and having no open space in the neighbourhood have been significantly correlated with higher temperatures. This risk will increase as the average and peak temperatures rise.

Urban flooding from a rising sea level and flooding from rivers will present an increasing risk to health. Health effects from flooding include drowning, injuries, infectious diseases, stress and loss of essential urban infrastructure and services. In terms of inequality in health, the effects of flooding can be particularly devastating to already vulnerable populations, such as children, older people, people with disabilities, ethnic minorities and those with low incomes. In addition, disadvantaged people may also live in areas that are more vulnerable to flooding.

1.6 Strategic focus

All these factors that affect disadvantaged people more than advantaged people and compound the effects of the social and economic determinants of health reflect the wider policy context in which land use, transport and development policies are shaped. Strategic decisions determining urban form affect the proximity of facilities, access to employment and income, access to high-quality green spaces and viable modes of transport and hence determine where people live and work and their mental well-being and physical health. The evidence demonstrates that health has a social gradient. People with better access to resources, services and life chances enjoy better health proportionately across that gradient.

A strategic and concerted focus on the social determinants of health means action across the life course to improve the conditions of daily life in which people are born, grow, live, work and age. This includes early child development and education, employment and working conditions, income and access to resources, training, people and places, transport and climate change and sustainability, with individuals and communities being empowered, thus enabling them to take greater control over their lives and to participate effectively, which enhances social cohesion and equity. These processes integrate the concepts of people and place. The framework for action *(6)* highlights the benefits of shifting to a more asset-based approach in engaging with communities and developing robust local partnerships orchestrated by local authorities with timely strategic documentation to deliver health equity (framework for action: sections 4.1.1, 4.1.2, 5.1, 5.2, 5.3.3 and 5.8.2).

Health and equity in health need to be assessed for both strategic plans and detailed neighbourhood decisions to ensure that the decisions made address inequities in health and do not introduce or further exacerbate them. Greater focus on the social determinants of health could be incorporated into strategic environmental assessment, health impact assessment and equity impact assessment. The framework for action *(6)* sets out key actions to effectively use data and incorporate this into health impact assessment to focus action and monitor outcomes (framework for action: sections 4.1, 5.1, 5.3.1, 5.3.3, 5.5, 5.7.4, 5.8.6 and 6.2).

Boxes 1 and 2 show examples of good practices.

Box 1. Reversing the trend by shaping places

Freiburg, Germany has pursued a committed, progressive and comprehensive land-use and transport strategy based on walking, cycling and public transport for the past three decades. People at all income levels have moved away from car use and have been given the freedom to travel around the city, giving equal access to jobs and housing in a healthier environment free from the dominance of cars. Recent urban development in the new neighbourhood of Vauban has established virtually car-free areas where children can play freely and safely, strengthening the community.

Box 2. Implementing a health in all policies approach in Slovenia

The operation of the school meals system is a good example of practical implementation, operating on the principle of health in all policies. This is particularly important because of the high employment levels of women in Slovenia. The system of well-organized school meals was upgraded during the implementation of the National Food and Nutrition Policy Programme 2005–2010. The system offers up to four meals a day for all children in primary schools. In secondary schools, the system offers students up to two organized meals or even more in exceptional cases. Virtually all primary schools and one quarter of all secondary schools have their own kitchens. Meals are prepared in accordance with the guidelines for a healthy diet that contain not only the physiological requirements but also instructions for preparing healthy meals and stressing the educational elements. One of the most important elements of the school meals is that they improve the social gradient. All children in both primary and secondary schools receive subsidized meals. About one third of the children, depending on socioeconomic status, receive meals free of charge.

Source: Buzeti et al. *(25)*.

2. How the report of the Commission on Social Determinants of Health and the strategic review of health inequalities in England post-2010 apply to urban settings

2.1 Introduction

This chapter summarizes the evidence and recommendations of the WHO Commission on Social Determinants of Health *(1)* and how they can be applied to urban settings in high- and medium-income countries. It also summarizes relevant evidence and recommendations from *Fair society, healthy lives: strategic review of health inequalities in England post-2010 (26)*, with a particular focus on the policy priority of creating and developing healthy and sustainable places and communities. It specifically addresses issues of active travel, access to quality space, social capital, place-shaping, sustainability and the built environment and integrating planning, transport, housing and environment and health in a whole-system process and partnership to address the wider social determinants of health.

The framework for action *(6)* provides guidance on developing collaborative partnership working and the creation of joint comprehensive strategies to secure political and stakeholder ownership (framework for action: sections 4.1, 4.3, 5.3.1, 5.3.3, 5.4, 5.7.4, 5.8.3, 6.1 and 6.2).

2.2 Commission on Social Determinants of Health

WHO commissioned the Commission on Social Determinants of Health (2005–2008), which had as its vision, "a world in which all people have the freedom to lead lives they have reason to value" *(1)*. Its aim was to catalyse a global movement to act on the social determinants of health to improve equity in health, the absence of avoidable, systematic differences in health between groups – identified by measures of socioeconomic position, occupation, education, geographical place of residence, sex, race and ethnicity, disability and intersections between groups (such as socioeconomic position and sex).

Differences in health in society are not dichotomized between people who are socially advantaged and disadvantaged but are frequently observed as gradients, with progressively worse health outcomes from the most advantaged to the least advantaged people in society. Life expectancy declines with every step down the income scale. The evidence on the social gradient in health *(1)* identifies that people who have higher socioeconomic status have a greater range of life chances and more opportunity to live flourishing lives and enjoy better health. Their health is graded by their socioeconomic position on the gradient. As a consequence, everyone other than those at the top of the gradient loses out.

The steepness of the gradient becomes critical, with health and social problems being less frequent in countries with less income inequality. Where income inequality is stronger, not only are the most disadvantaged people most affected but the overall burden is higher than in more equal societies *(27)*.

The Commission conceptualized the social determinants of health as the conditions in which people live their daily lives and the structural influences on these conditions that ultimately reflect the distribution of power and resources within and between countries. The Commission collected, collated and analysed evidence from around the world about the social determinants of health and the policies and programmes that affect them. Based on this evidence, the Commission set forward recommendations for action on the social determinants of health with the aim of encouraging countries, global institutions and national and international organizations to take action to improve population health, improve the distribution of health and reduce disadvantage due to ill health *(28)*. Simply put, the Commission concluded that societal inequities in health arise from social inequalities. Reducing inequities in health and thereby improving overall population health requires action to address the processes that promote relative disadvantage and social exclusion by building a fairer society.

The Commission proposed three principles of action to tackle inequities in health:
- improve the conditions of daily life – the circumstances in which people are born, grow, live, work and age;
- tackle the inequitable distribution of power, money and resources – the structural drivers of these conditions of daily life – globally, nationally and locally; and
- measure the problem, evaluate action, expand the knowledge base, develop a workforce that is trained in the social determinants of health and raise public awareness about the social determinants of health.

Within this framework, the Commission made recommendations for action in the areas of: early child development and education, the built environment and sustainable development, employment arrangements and work conditions, social protection, health care systems, health equity in all policies, fair financing, market responsibility, gender equity, political empowerment and voice, global governance and monitoring, training and research.

All these areas for action are relevant to urban settings, and many fall outside the health sector. Addressing the social determinants of health most effectively requires the health sector to work with other sectors at every level, local and national, both within government and within the wider society.

2.2.1 Measuring the problem

Data on mortality and morbidity by socioeconomic group, sex, ethnicity and race, geographical area of residence or within local areas by scales of deprivation and data on the distribution of social determinants of health underpin advocacy and action on social determinants of health. Establishing national systems for measuring and monitoring equity in health and routinely collecting data on the social determinants of health from which inequities in health arise are fundamental to the process of developing national and local strategies to reduce inequities in health. The framework for action *(6)* discusses issues of using data effectively to develop robust strategies and monitor progress on inequities in health (framework for action: sections 4.1.1, 5.1, 5.2, 5.3.1, 5.5, 5.8.6 and 6.3).

2.2.2 Health equity in all policies – working across sectors

The Commission's recommendations are based on the understanding that policy in every sector of government can potentially affect health and inequities in health. Although health may not be the explicit focus in many policy areas, unless the potential effects of these policy areas on health and equity in health are considered, opportunities will probably be missed for both reducing gradients in health and creating side benefits for other outcomes. Coordinated action between sectors has the potential to contribute to significant health gains. Health equity impact assessment of all policies and programmes, as part of the process of health impact assessment, needs to become a routine step in developing policy.

Intersectoral action requires building effective partnerships, nationally and locally, across government departments, agencies and institutions, the third sector and, where appropriate, the private sector. Activities at the local level that often facilitate active public participation in community planning and programme development are crucial to addressing inequities in health. Such initiatives need to be supported by a funding mechanism and accountability structure that respond to local needs. Framing this issue in terms that bring together the interests of all partners is important in initiating partnerships across sectors that have differing organizational cultures and practices (Box 3).

2.2.3 Global governance

Factors at the global level, such as global financial markets, trade and the changing climate, that lie outside the regulatory power of one country acting alone and require cooperation between the world's countries influence the social determinants of health that operate at the local level through the conditions in which people live their daily lives. Low- and middle-income countries and people with low income in all countries suffer disproportionately from the hazards associated with the processes of globalization, while the people with high income globally take a greater share of the benefits. The Commission on Social Determinants of Health recommended that the institutions and processes of global governance be reformed so that all countries participate fairly and are equitably represented and that equity in health should become a global development goal.

2.2.4 Political empowerment and voice

All the Commission's recommendations emphasize the importance of political empowerment at all levels of decision-making. Fair representation of individual and community concerns and interests in the processes of decision-making at the local level underpins the development of equity in health. Many mechanisms for public participation in local decision-making are evident across the European Region. Nevertheless, many mechanisms for public participation in decision-making could be radically improved and the social determinants of health could be addressed.

2.2.5 Gender equity

Achieving gender equity in health implies eliminating differences between men and women that are avoidable and unnecessary and therefore unfair. Men and women have traditionally occupied different social roles in most societies. These confer differences in living and working conditions. Progress towards gender equity has varied considerably both between and within countries. Participation by women and men in national and local government continues to be highly imbalanced in many countries.

To promote gender equity, the Commission urged countries and organizations to address gender biases in the structures of society, through legislation, by using mechanisms at national and local level to ana-

---

Box 3. Building the case for intersectoral action

▶ Building on public concern for the health and well-being of a disadvantaged group

▶ Using political champions to advocate for intersectoral action

▶ Framing the issue in a way that all sectors can recognize

▶ Building on international leadership

▶ Creating a platform for researchers

▶ Building on concerns about the need to use scarce resources more efficiently

▶ Acknowledging the limitations of previous approaches, especially those involving sectors working alone

▶ Taking advantage of political transitions to reassess roles and begin to work better together

▶ Building consensus via shared gatherings, such as conferences or community meetings

Source: Peake et al. *(28)*.

lyse and act on the gender implications of policies, programmes and institutional arrangements and by changing the indicators used to measure a country's economic performance to include the contributions of caring for home and family and voluntary work.

2.2.6 Market responsibility

Markets bring great benefits such as new technologies, goods and services that in many cases improve the conditions of daily life, but they may also have negative effects. The aims of pro-equity policies are to ensure a more equitable distribution of high-quality services and resources fundamental to health and to ensure effective regulation of products, activities and conditions that tend to damage health or lead to inequities in health. Much of this action must take place at the national and supranational levels. However, local government is responsible for regulating the spatial distribution of many goods and services, such as food retailers, licensed premises, recreational amenities and facilities and education and health facilities.

2.2.7 Early childhood development

The early years of life are a critical period for child development in the linked areas of social, emotional, language, cognitive and physical development. Early child development in these domains strongly influences the subsequent life course through the attainment of skills, education and employment opportunities and effects on health outcomes. Evidence shows that investing in early child development has the potential to be a powerful equalizer, with interventions having the largest effects among the most deprived children (29).

For older children of primary and secondary school age, attention to social and emotional learning as well as language, cognitive and physical development can potentially improve school attendance, educational attainment and health.

The Commission called for a comprehensive approach to the early years and education, starting before birth. This requires collaboration between service providers and participation in decision-making by user groups, including parents and children, to ensure the appropriate delivery of high-quality, effective services to mothers and children at the local level.

2.2.8 The built environment and sustainable development

As indicated in Chapter 1, the built environment affects health through the extent to which it helps or hinders access to goods, services and the natural environment and promotes social cohesion and physical and mental well-being. Good governance at the local level is crucial in improving health and reducing inequities in health. Further, evidence is growing that interventions in the built environment that improve health may have side benefits for the environment by reducing emissions of greenhouse gases. The Urban Settings Knowledge Network of the Commission (8) identified key steps in developing interventions for equity in health in urban settings (Box 4).

Box 4. Developing healthy urban governance interventions

▶ Community organization and participation for defining the problems and empowering the community

▶ Identifying interventions based on scientific and technical evidence

▶ Ensuring the availability of financial resources to draw on for implementation

▶ Implementing for and with the community

▶ Monitoring and evaluating the health and social effects

Source: Knowledge Network on Urban Settings of the Commission on Social Determinants of Health (8).

2.3 The strategic review of health inequalities in England post-2010

The 2010 review of health inequalities in England post-2010 *(26)* gathered together the best available evidence on inequalities in health. It calculated that, if everyone in England had the same death rates as the most advantaged people, those who are currently dying prematurely as a result of inequalities in health would have enjoyed a total of 1.3 million to 2.5 million extra years of life. They would, in addition, have had a further 2.8 million years free of limiting illness or disability. This illness accounts for productivity losses estimated at £31 billion to £33 billion per year, lost taxes and higher welfare payments in the range of £20 billion to £32 billion per year and additional National Health Service health care costs well in excess of £5.5 billion per year *(26)*.

A substantial proportion of these individual, social and economic costs of inequalities in health fall on the cities where most of the population lives. In the current economic climate, these inequalities and their associated costs are likely to increase. It is therefore even more important that local government do everything in its power to reduce inequalities in health both now and for the longer term.

This section explores these social determinants, alongside the key evidence and recommendations from the Marmot Review that relate to people and place and on which urban local authorities need to act in addressing inequalities in health (Fig. 2).

Fair society, healthy lives (26) emphasizes that the social determinants of health have different effects at different stages of the life course. When both people and place factors are considered, the issues that need to be tackled at various stages of the life course also need to be considered.

Disadvantage starts before birth and accumulates throughout life. A people and place focus on addressing the social determinants of health in a scaled up and systematic response is needed to reduce the steepness

Fig. 2. A life-course approach

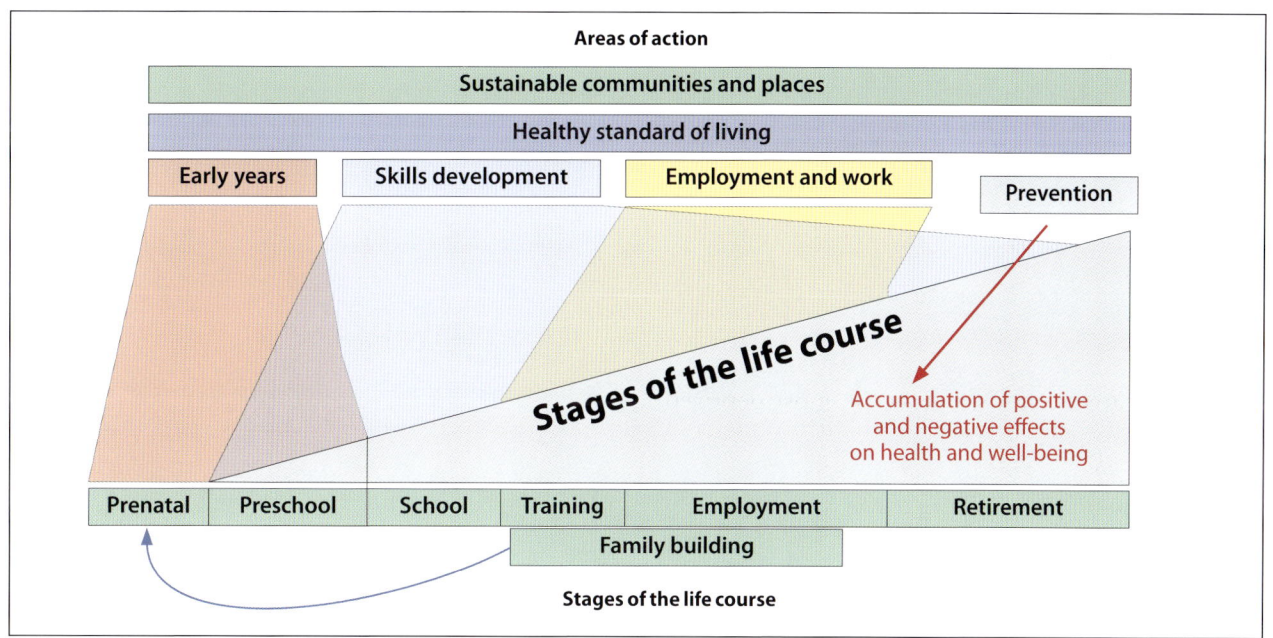

Source: *Fair society, healthy lives: strategic review of health inequalities in England post-2010 (26)*. Reproduced with permission.

of the social gradient in health and close the health divide *(6)*.

2.3.1 Issues related to people

As stated in the report *(26)*, numerous social determinants affect people differentially and cumulatively across the life course, both as individuals and social groups. These include early childhood experiences, educational outcomes, employment and quality of work, income and health behaviour.

2.3.1.1 Early childhood experiences

A substantial body of evidence shows that experiences in the first few years of life have a profound effect on our health and development throughout the life course *(1)*. Early childhood lays the foundations for key aspects of human development – physical, intellectual and emotional.

2.3.1.2. Educational outcomes

The early cognitive and non-cognitive skills developed combined with numerous other individual, family, school and environmental factors affect educational achievement and social skills, which in turn are key predictors of subsequent outcomes, including physical and mental health, income, employment and quality of life. Educational attainment has a strong social gradient across the European Region and is significantly correlated with health.

2.3.1.3 Employment and quality of work

Being in good employment protects health. Conversely, unemployment contributes to poor health. Getting people into work is therefore critically important in reducing inequalities in health. However, work needs to be good – both sustainable and offering a minimum level of quality. This includes not only a decent living wage but also being managed well, with low levels of work-related stress and a high level of job control, opportunities for in-work development, the flexibility to enable people to balance work and family life and protection from other adverse work conditions that can damage health.

2.3.1.4 Income

Good employment is associated with adequate income levels, but the extent to which people have a level of income to enable them to live healthily also depends on access to fair and adequate social protection systems.

The Marmot Review *(26)* recommended a minimum income for healthy living. The minimum income for healthy living is calculated contextually, varying according to the family circumstances of individuals and within and between countries. It includes the level of income needed for adequate diet, physical activity, housing, social interaction, participation, transport, health care and personal hygiene.

2.3.1.5 Health behaviour

The European health report 2009 (7) identifies seven individual-level factors responsible for about 60% of the burden of disease in the WHO European Region: high blood pressure, tobacco use, harmful use of alcohol, high serum cholesterol, overweight, unhealthy diet and insufficient physical activity.

They tend to be more prevalent among people with less education, lower occupational status and lower income. They include health-damaging behaviour that often reflects or is linked to coping mechanisms for people in materially deprived circumstances.

2.3.2 Place issues

Place also affects health and inequities in health, often interacting with the issues related to people described above. Key place factors include the environment and neighbourhoods and communities.

2.3.2.1 The environment

Environmental issues are a common and growing health concern across Europe. The primary factors affecting health are access to safe drinking-water and sanitation, air quality, occupational safety and injuries. More than 1.7 million deaths per year (18% of all annual deaths) in the European Region are attributable to environmental factors. The environment accounts for an estimated one third of the total burden of disease among people 0–19 years old. The burden of disease caused by known environmental factors varies up to fourfold between countries *(7)*.

2.3.2.2 Neighbourhoods and communities

Some environmental factors affect whole countries, whereas others are largely confined to or have the greatest effect on cities or specific neighbourhoods. The physical and social characteristics of communities and the degree to which they enable and promote healthy behaviour contribute to social inequalities in health (see Chapter 1).

2.3.2.3 Recommendations from the Marmot Review

Reducing inequalities in health requires action on six key policy objectives *(26)*:
- "give every child the best start in life";
- "enable all children, young people and adults to maximize their capabilities and have control over their lives";
- "create fair employment and good work for all";
- "ensure [a] healthy standard of living for all";
- "create and develop healthy and sustainable places and communities"; and
- "strengthen the role and impact of ill health prevention".

2.3.2.3.1 *"Give every child the best start in life"*

Action to reduce inequalities in health must start before birth and be followed throughout the life of the child. Only then can the close links between early disadvantage and poor outcomes throughout life be broken. Reducing inequalities in early child development by giving every child the best start in life is crucial.

This involves action to reduce inequalities in the early development of physical and emotional health and cognitive, linguistic and social skills and to build the resilience and well-being of young children across the social gradient. Good evidence supports increasing children's access to positive early experiences to reduce inequalities in health. Later interventions are important too but are considerably less effective without good early foundations *(30)*. Specific evidence-informed priorities include the following.

- Maternal health should be promoted through high-quality maternity services, giving priority to pre- and postnatal interventions that reduce adverse outcomes of pregnancy and infancy. Maternal and fetal nutrition, birth weight and growth by age one year all predict later adult health.
- Ongoing support should be provided to parents to achieve progressive improvements in early childhood development. This needs to include paid parental leave, support for families through parenting programmes and outreach services and supporting the transition into school.
- High-quality preschool childcare and education should be delivered to meet needs across the social gradient. Good international evidence indicates the effectiveness of early-childhood care and education programmes, which have been shown to especially benefit disadvantaged children.

Meeting these priorities clearly requires funding from national governments. The Marmot Review *(26)* recommended an increase in the proportion of overall expenditure allocated to the early years along with steps to ensure that spending on early-childhood development is focused progressively across the social gradient. National governments make important decisions to increase overall expenditure. However, in most countries, local government has a critical contribution to make to setting priorities and shaping and implementing local provision.

2.3.2.3.2 "Enable all children, young people and adults to maximize their capabilities and have control over their lives"

Maintaining the reduction in inequality across the gradient that follows from appropriate investment in the early years requires a sustained commitment to children and young people through the years of education.

Central to this is acquiring cognitive and non-cognitive skills, which are strongly associated with both educational achievement and many other outcomes, including better employment, income and physical and mental health. Specific evidence-informed priorities include the following.

Social inequalities in the acquisition of cognitive and life skills should be reduced. Early-childhood care and education can build good foundations for children, but these need to be followed through into full-time education. Action can include programmes to increase school readiness for children from disadvantaged backgrounds and to improve the basic skills of parents and encourage their involvement in their child's education *(31)*.

Strong links should be built between schools, families and communities, and a whole-child approach to education should be taken. Schools can play an important role in communities, and this may be especially important in deprived urban areas, where schools may be a valuable community resource for extended childcare and adult learning *(32)*.

Good evidence, especially from the Nordic countries, indicates the value of having a school-based workforce working across the school–home boundaries *(33)*.

Access to and the use of quality life-long learning opportunities across the social gradient should be increased. Education does not just take place in school, and it does not stop once people leave school. Ensuring that young adults have easily accessible support and advice on life skills, training and employment opportunities is especially important. Given the ageing population in many parts of the European Region, another need is to ensure that people can maintain their capacity to remain in the workforce for longer.

2.3.2.3.3 "Create fair employment and good work for all"

High-quality work benefits physical and mental health, and unemployment, especially long-term unemployment, is associated with adverse health outcomes. The evidence suggests that policies to reduce the social gradient in employment and working conditions should be focused on three interrelated policy objectives: to improve access to good work and reduce long-term unemployment across the social gradient; to make it easier for people who are disadvantaged in the labour market to obtain and keep work; and to improve the quality of work across the social gradient.

Specific evidence-informed priorities include the following.

Active labour market programmes should be implemented to integrate unemployed people into work rather than simply providing passive income support to people without work. Various types of active labour market programmes have become a major feature of international labour market policy and social development interventions. Countries in the Organisation for Economic Co-operation and Development have especially extensive experience in active labour market programmes, often targeted at people who are long-term unemployed, workers in low-income families and specific groups with labour-market disadvantages.

The evidence suggests that such programmes can succeed in getting people into jobs and contribute to increasing income among recipients, although they have been most effective when combined with other fiscal and benefits measures to make work pay. Some evidence also suggests that participating in active labour market programmes can improve health, despite material circumstances remaining poor, via psychosocial mechanisms such as increased social contact, social support and generating feelings of control and self-worth.

Safe, secure and fairly paid work and healthy work–life balances should be developed, and measures should be implemented to improve the quality of work across the social gradient. Employers are responsible for complying with legal requirements and monitoring and controlling the working environment. Successful implementation requires the laws to be sufficiently robust, the enforcement agencies to be adequately resourced and the legal framework to be sufficiently clear to enable prosecution to succeed. Undertaking unambiguous and comprehensive risk assessment is an essential prerequisite.

Improving the psychosocial quality of working environments is important. Lack of control and lack of reward at work have been shown to be critical determinants of a variety of stress-related disorders and to be more prevalent among people with lower occupational status. Focusing interventions around these dimensions by ensuring clear leadership and good stress management policies in the workplace and targeting less privileged groups within the workforce is a high priority.

Steps also need to be taken to adapt working hours and practices to increase access to good work for groups who are disadvantaged in the labour market. Action could include improving the flexibility of working practices and retirement age and encouraging and providing incentives for employers to create or adapt jobs that are suitable for lone parents, caregivers and people with mental and physical health problems.

2.3.2.3.4 "Ensure [a] healthy standard of living for all"

Having enough money to lead a healthy life is central to reducing inequalities in health. Policies are needed that address the situation of the people with the lowest income and ensure that the fiscal and social protection systems are not regressive, perpetuating inequality.

Specific evidence-informed priorities include establishing a minimum income for healthy living for people of all ages and reducing the social gradient in the standard of living through progressive tax policy and other fiscal policies. The absence of health needs in the existing minimum income requirements sparked the development of the concept of a minimum income for healthy living *(34)*. This income level covers a healthy diet, the costs of physical activity and costs related to social integration and support networks, such as those for telephone, television and presents, and takes account of social norms and expectations.

A minimum income for healthy living would improve the standard of living for those with low incomes. It would ensure that everyone would receive an appropriate income for their stage in the life course and would reduce overall levels of poverty as well as child poverty.

Social protection schemes are designed to smooth income flows across the life course and act as a buffer against the times when people have difficulty in obtaining and maintaining secure employment or adequate pay. Ideally, a social protection system offers people the opportunities to maintain a decent standard of living while:

- assisting and encouraging people to remain in work when they experience poor health or other life-changing events such as divorce or new caring responsibilities;
- facilitating the transition into work or self-employment as people's health improves or other responsibilities change;
- enabling and providing incentives for people to move into retirement at a pace that reflects their health and wider capabilities;
- creating opportunities for people to prepare for alternative careers through access to training and upgrading of skills; and
- providing the support families require when bringing up their children.

However, most current social protection systems fail to fulfil the above criteria.

The available evidence indicates that more generous social protection systems improve population health outcomes and increase life expectancy. Welfare policies may also differ with regard to their ability to buffer against the adverse health effects of economic crises and substantial job instability.

Some evidence indicates that social inequalities in health have tended to remain stable in Nordic countries during periods of economic recession, whereas they are widening in other countries in the European Region with both more liberal and conservative policies.

2.3.2.3.5 "Create and develop healthy and sustainable places and communities"

As indicated in Chapter 1, the neighbourhoods and communities in which people live influence their health and well-being. In addition to physical places, the communities and social networks to which individuals belong over their life course also significantly affect health and inequalities in health. The links connecting people within communities – often described as social or community capital – can bring a range of benefits. Social capital can provide a source of resilience, a buffer against high risks of poor health, through social support and connections that help people find work or get through economic and other difficulties. The extent of people's participation in their communities and the added control over their lives that this brings can potentially contribute to their psychosocial well-being and thereby to other health outcomes.

The creation of healthy, sustainable places and communities should go hand in hand with the mitigation of climate change and have a shared policy agenda. Specific evidence-informed priorities that both reduce inequalities in health and mitigate climate change include the following.

Active transport should be increased across the social gradient. Active transport can contribute substantially to overall physical health and mental well-being. Improving active transport probably requires incentives to increase levels and investment to improve safety. Traffic-calming measures have an important role. Five to seven times as many children are killed by cars in the poor areas of cities in Great Britain than in more affluent areas.

Access to high-quality open and green spaces across the social gradient should be improved. Green space and green infrastructure improve mental and physical health and have been shown to reduce inequalities in health *(22)*. Simply providing more green spaces is not enough – attention also needs to be paid to their design and quality.

The food environment in local areas should be improved. This involves addressing the accessibility of affordable and nutritious food that is sustainably produced, processed and delivered. Internationally, studies show that price is the greatest motivating factor in food choice among low-income groups. In the United States, reducing prices has increased the sales of low-fat foods and fruit and vegetables. The availability of healthy food, especially fresh produce, is often worse in deprived areas because of the mix of shops that tend to locate in these neighbourhoods.

The quality and energy efficiency of housing across the social gradient should be improved. Poor control of heat (cold in winter or hot in summer) causes deaths and other adverse health events among older people and people with pre-existing health problems. Poor housing quality can contribute to developing chronic conditions among children.

The planning, transport, housing, environment and health systems should be integrated to address the social determinants of health in local areas. As indicated in Chapter 1, the effects of the factors described above on health are compounded by features controlled through the planning of the built environment, such as road design, lighting and access to transport, amenities and other facilities. These in turn reflect the wider policy context in which land-use, transport and development policies are shaped. Chapter 3 discusses this further.

Locally developed and evidence-informed community regeneration programmes that remove barriers to community participation and action and reduce social isolation should be supported. Community or social capital is shaped both by the ability of communities to define and organize themselves and by the extent to which national and local organizations seek to involve and empower communities. Disadvantaged areas are frequently described in terms of need, problems, deficiencies, deprivation and health-damaging behaviour. A more asset-based approach that engages citizens as co-producers of health and well-being shifts the emphasis away from professionally driven, top-down models and solutions to supporting communities to take control, building local networks that sustain individual and collective well-being and avoid stress, depression and social isolation.

2.3.2.3.6 "Strengthen the role and impact of ill health prevention"

As discussed above, many of the key types of health behaviour and lifestyles that promote disease follow a social gradient: smoking, obesity, lack of physical activity and unhealthy diet. Reducing inequalities in health requires focusing on these types of health behaviour and addressing the wider determinants of health.

Health systems have traditionally been considered responsible for preventing ill health, but tackling the social determinants of health requires efforts by a wide range of stakeholders. Local and national decisions made in schools, the workplace, at home and in government services can all potentially help or hinder the prevention of ill health. Partnerships between primary health care, local authorities and nongovernmental organizations can deliver effective universal and targeted preventive interventions and have important benefits. Investing in preventing ill health, if implemented effectively, can improve health and life expectancy and reduce spending over the long term. Although the evidence base on the effectiveness of public health interventions to reduce inequalities in health is growing, it remains modest. Advantaged population groups more frequently take up some population-wide interventions, such as screening programmes, potentially widening inequalities in health. People who are more advantaged and people who already have positive attitudes towards health more successfully adopt policies to prevent ill health aimed at changing individual behaviour, such as that related to smoking, alcohol, diet and physical activity. Both population-wide and individually targeted interventions therefore need to be proportionately targeted across the social gradient if they are to reduce inequalities in health effectively.

Specific evidence-informed priorities seek to increase the proportion of investment allocated to preventing ill health across the social gradient, including reducing smoking and harmful alcohol use.

2.3.2.3.7 Role of local government in developing healthy, sustainable places and communities and in preventing ill health

Local government has a clear role in place-shaping local neighbourhoods and communities. Urban planners are critical in this regard and need to be strongly aware of the potential of urban design to both increase and decrease inequalities in health. However, the whole of local government, business and local communities themselves need to have a wider partnership approach. Local government has a specific role in:
- identifying population needs, including collecting information from communities to inform the design of neighbourhoods and the local development of services and facilities, including a range of data concerning gender and socioeconomic variables,

the effects on equity in health and regular and robust monitoring of progress as set out in the framework for action *(6)* (framework for action: sections 4.1, 5.3.1, 5.3.3, 5.6 and 5.8.6);
- promoting and supporting communities in participating in co-producing, directing and controlling local services and/or interventions and building health, well-being and resilience in a more asset-based approach to community engagement, as explored in the framework for action *(6)* (framework for action: sections 4.1.1, 4.1.2, 5.1, 5.2 and 5.3.3);
- developing social capital by enhancing community empowerment to develop relationships of trust, reciprocity and exchange within communities and encouraging local action to challenge the material circumstances of neighbourhoods in an approach related to people, place and process outline in the framework for action *(6)* (framework for action: sections 4.1, 5.1, 5.2, 5.5, 6.1 and 6.2);
- assessing the effects of urban planning on health and inequalities in health both in relation to design and regenerating existing neighbourhoods in place-making initiatives, and building understanding and awareness of how policies and initiatives on inequities in health and the overall benefits to society create new opportunities for engagement and ownership across a range of stakeholders (framework for action: sections 4.1, 5.1, 5.7.4 and 6.2);
- giving priority to access to green spaces and community safety in spatial planning and introducing evidence-informed measures to reduce road traffic and the speed of motor vehicles, such as traffic-calming, speed limits and home zones;
- ensuring that fuel efficiency is a key priority in both new housing developments and refurbishments of older housing stock;
- using local regulatory mechanisms to limit the number of retail fast food outlets, especially in deprived areas;
- giving priority to evidence-informed preventive strategies, including targeted smoking cessation and using regulatory mechanisms to control alcohol sales; and
- acting as an exemplary employer and using commissioning and contracting powers to improve working conditions within the local area.

3. Local government and the social determinants of health: an overview of policy and practice in the WHO European Region

3.1 Introduction
This chapter considers the role of local government across the WHO European Region beginning with England and initiatives taken to address inequities in health during the past decade and then presenting the outcome of work commissioned to review the role of local government in relation to the social determinants of health across the European Region using examples in Denmark, Latvia, the Netherlands, Spain and Sweden. Overall, this provides a wide perspective of local government within various settings and cultures and supports thematic evaluation.

3.2 Approaches to tackling inequalities in health in England
The health of the population of the United Kingdom has improved substantially during the past decade, but inequalities in health have widened. The policy debate in the United Kingdom has two major approaches, one short term and the other longer term.

In the short term, the Department of Health focuses on removing the inequalities "tail" – the most disadvantaged quartile of areas. The nine national support teams are working closely with these localities (the 78 "spearhead" areas, which are mostly industrial cities and towns). Their aim is to help them make better use of what is known to work well and to encourage them to act urgently, on a large scale and with more systematic application. The approach is saving lives and has the potential to save many more, but it will not be sufficient by itself to remove the health risks in the first place.

A longer-term approach looking at the social gradient and the causes of the causes of inequalities in health is needed, and this can be constructed using the framework of the strategic review of health inequalities in England (see Chapter 2). The recently published London Health Inequalities Strategy *(35)* illustrates well what can be done to shape strategies to deal with the wider determinants of health even during recession and public sector retrenchment. There is a strong business case for all local councils to invest in health and identifying the economic gain alongside the health gain *(36)*.

3.2.1 England's local councils and health
Several features of local government in England are important in relation to the social determinants of health.
- Policy-makers prefer "healthy communities" to "healthy cities, towns and villages", which is more commonly used in the European Region.
- England has a strong central state, with a recent history of firm direction and performance management for improving health and local government. The depth and intensity of central performance review has led to tensions between the national and local governments. The performance management regime included regular and detailed reporting against targets and inspection of services by public regulatory authorities.
- Local intersectoral partnerships for improving health are important, especially between the local government and its local primary care National Health Service trust. Joint work between health and local government had been a feature of the local landscape for more than two decades, but progress towards better outcomes has been slow. The

introduction of community strategies as statements of local needs and aspirations together with multi-agency and multidisciplinary local strategic partnerships established after 2000 reinforced joint partnership working. This may have led to stronger strategic alliances and more productive joint working between health agencies and local government through joint strategic needs assessments required by the Local Government and Public Involvement Health Act (2007). The aim was to jointly assess the current and future health and well-being needs of the local population to inform local priorities for action and local targets for achievement, leading to joint commissioning policies to improve outcomes and reduce inequalities in health. More recently, through what are called "total place" pilots, efforts have been made to map all the public expenditure being channelled into a local government area and to develop more productive jointly funded programmes. These aim to improve quality and effectiveness while reducing costs.

An important turning point in rebuilding the confidence of local government in England was the publication of *National prosperity, local choice and civic engagement (37)*, which attempted to define the purpose of local councils for the 21st century. The approach was expressed in the term place shaping. This can be understood as applying legal powers to promote economic, social and environmental well-being of people and places. Place shaping is the key community leadership role for local councils and inherently includes addressing issues related to people and places in the context of the social determinants of health across the social gradient.

3.2.2 Progress so far

Local councils in England from across the political spectrum have increasingly sought to take steps to improve the health of local people and reduce inequalities in health. By providing leadership, engaging in intersectoral partnerships and directing council services, they are in a key position to mobilize action across the sectors to tackle inequalities in health and developing people, places and process. However, little evidence indicates that local partnerships have produced better health outcomes for local populations or reduced inequalities in health *(38)*.

Nevertheless, health and well-being remain central themes for local government. Most local councils are trying hard to promote healthy living across the life course. This is illustrated by the councils supporting early interventions through the Sure Start and other Healthy Schools initiatives.

Councils have other less well-known areas of activity that have considerable importance for health. One is regulation, which is often ignored in accounts of the local government contribution to health but supports better health for local people. Another important area of council involvement is the work of overview and scrutiny committees for health, which have a responsibility for reviewing inequalities in health and public health as well as local health services.

3.2.3 Spatial planning and health in England's councils

Local councils arguably can have their most important long-term effects on health through the decisions they take about spatial planning. The Commission for Architecture and the Built Environment *(39)* described the built environment as the "foundation asset of our health". Planning decisions, transport, housing, public spaces and service and flooding have major effects on health and well-being *(40)*. Poor transport planning, for example, can lead to road crashes, noise and air pollution and sedentary lifestyles. Further, roads that are difficult to cross reduce social contact, harm community cohesion and deepen personal isolation. Inadequate housing and poor neighbourhood planning expose people to damp and cold, accidents and falls, noise pollution, road safety problems and problems with crime and community cohesion. Feeling unsafe is often associated with poorer health, whereas the provision of space that was perceived as safe increases levels of exercise and self-reported emotional well-being *(41)*. Local councils should work to increase the amount of high-quality, well-supervised open space and create local playgrounds in every neighbourhood.

3.2.4 Healthy lives, healthy people

The recent public health white paper *Healthy lives, healthy people: our strategy for public health in England (42)* proposes shifting the lead responsibility for public health to local councils by April 2013 and creating a national public health service, Public Health England. It also adopts a life-course approach, accepting that the social conditions in which people live drive inequalities in health while acknowledging the social gradient in health. Given this analysis, local government is seen as the appropriate lead organization to orchestrate local action to address inequalities in health.

A report by the Department of Health *(43)* summed up the challenges as "much achieved: more to do". Although life expectancy has risen for each social group and most areas, the social gradient has persisted, with no reduction in the gap between the bottom and top.

National targets and a range of national policy initiatives have reflected awareness of inequalities in health. However, attempts to reduce inequalities in health have not systematically addressed the social determinants of health and have relied increasingly on tackling more proximal causes through behaviour change programmes.

Perceptions that health services are solely responsible for health have hampered progress. Although health care contributes substantially in tackling access to services, the key drivers are the conditions in which people are born, grow, live, work and age. Local government has increasingly taken responsibilities for health and health inequalities seriously and led partnership working with National Health Service primary care trusts and other key stakeholders. This is consistent with the proposals in *Healthy lives, healthy people (42)* of strengthening the responsibilities of local councils to secure the health and well-being of their local population. A framework for delivery through local partnerships will remain a feature combined with joint strategic needs assessments. This system is being radically reformed in a context of severe public-sector spending cuts, which threaten services and significantly challenge local government.

3.3 Overview of policy and practice in Denmark, Latvia, the Netherlands, Spain and Sweden

3.3.1 Structure and method

This section extends an overview of the work of local governments in tackling inequities in health in the European Region. Local government authorities from Denmark, Latvia, the Netherlands, Spain and Sweden were selected for in-depth interviews. The purpose of the interviews was to explore in greater detail the political and fiscal context of local government in different parts of the European Region, to draw out the practical experience of local government in its action on the social determinants of health and inequities in health and to gather intelligence on the specific experience of implementing initiatives at the local level. In addition, work was commissioned to draw on existing academic and policy literature.

The countries chosen represent a wide variety of policy and governance contexts in the European Region and different levels of national income, life expectancy and health outcome. The local authorities were identified through the membership network of the European Health Management Association; they include both subnational regions and cities to explore the diversity of forms and scope of local government. The aim was not specifically to identify cities that are leading this agenda, especially at the international level; regions and cities that are members of the WHO European Healthy Cities Network and other leading-edge initiatives were therefore not included. The cities interviewed were Maastricht, the Netherlands, Aarhus, Denmark and Jurmula, Latvia; the regions interviewed were Aragon, Spain (most important city: Zaragoza) and Västra Götaland, Sweden (most important city: Göteborg).

The method used was a structured interview with policy staff from the city or region. Interviewees expressed views on behalf of their city or region. A blinded reviewer from the countries' local government associations then checked the information.

This section has four parts. The first describes the contextual frameworks of local government in each country as they affect the social determinants of health and inequities in health, including the legal and fiscal framework, political leadership and recent changes where relevant. The second section elaborates the activities of local authorities and the domains in which they are carrying out work that aims to explicitly address the social determinants of health and inequities in health. The topics discussed in this section, chosen for their potential effects on social determinants of health and inequities in health, are:
- the development of children and young people – action area 5 in the report of the Commission on Social Determinants of Health (1);
- employment and a good work balance – action area 7;
- older people – action area 8; and
- the development of healthy and sustainable places and communities – action area 6.

The third section focuses specifically on the experience of local authorities in implementing initiatives tackling the social determinants of health, including barriers and factors for successfully implementing initiatives. The final section concludes by drawing out potential policy implications from the interviews.

3.3.2 Terms

All the interviewees used the social determinants of health and action on inequities in health interchangeably. In addition, the interviewees generally assumed that action on inequities in health is also interchangeable with targeting vulnerable groups rather than action across the gradient. The social determinants of health and inequities in health are therefore used together in this account as shorthand for approaches in local government that focus on the social determinants of health and recognize their potential effects on inequities in health. Whether interventions have been specifically targeted or have been designed to have effects across the gradient has been explored and highlighted on a case-by-case basis.

3.3.3 Political and fiscal context for tackling the social determinants of health and inequities in health in local government

Identifying the political and fiscal context to local government and the similarities and differences across the European Region is central to understanding the role of local government and its potential effects on the social determinants of health and inequities in health in the European Region. Indeed, the Assembly of European Regions has mapped the various subnational structures of local government in the European Region (44,45) and shown that the situation is complex.

To explore the various political and fiscal contexts in greater depth, the interviews explicitly covered countries with both strong regional governments (Spain and Sweden) and those with strong municipal governments (Denmark, Latvia and the Netherlands). This section describes the specific legal context or responsibility for tackling the social determinants of health or reducing inequities in health for each of the five countries. If such responsibility exists and if it is backed up by an identified or separate funding source, this has also been identified. In addition, this section explores how the responsibility for tackling the social determinants of health is apportioned and whether it is considered primarily a concern for the health system or for local government, either regional or municipal. Since the factors influencing the determinants of health are complex, this section also considers whether and how action is coordinated across different organizations, sectors and tiers within the system.

3.3.3.1 Denmark

In Denmark, a reform of local government structure in 2007 changed the distribution of responsibilities within the health care system. Local government (98 amalgamated municipalities, reduced from 271) is mainly responsible for health promotion, nursing homes and services for groups with special needs, and the five newly created administrative regions run and own hospitals and care centres and are responsible for primary and secondary curative health care *(46)*. Both these levels of government have earmarked revenue sources.

The 2007 reforms made tackling inequities in health and the social determinants of health a municipal task. The municipality interviewed said that there has been increased focus on these topics since 2007.

This has also been backed up by policy changes, with the result that many municipalities have developed policy plans on how they will approach inequities in health. According to the interviewee, these changes have had direct positive effects: "The reform of Denmark's local government structure certainly had an impact, as people are more aware that health is a new focus of the municipalities. We know that the level of information on health care and healthy living has increased."

Denmark's municipalities also have a financial incentive to focus on social determinants of health and inequities in health. With municipalities paying for up to 30% of Denmark's total health care budget, this has increasingly become an incentive to work on upstream health promotion interventions in an attempt to limit expenditure on the larger and more expensive curative health care system. There are also budgets earmarked for health promotion and funds for supporting deprived groups, such as people who use illicit drugs.

The municipality interviewed also stressed the importance of partnerships in moving health and inequalities in health onto the agenda of other policy areas. Stakeholders from outside the health system that are currently engaged include housing associations and schools. According to the respondent: "The importance of tackling inequities in health and the social determinants of health is slowly diffusing to other non-health areas. In Aarhus, for example, health impact assessment has become part of planning in urban governance."

3.3.3.2 Latvia

In Latvia, local government gained an important role in financing and providing health care services in 1993 as the result of an extensive decentralization process. The financial processes were centralized once again in 1997, while the provision of health services gradually became more independent from local government. Although local government is still formally responsible for primary care and hospitals, centres and hospitals have become mainly self-managing actors, leaving local government responsible for health promotion and providing services for older people and homeless people. Latvia's municipalities are legally required to provide a minimum housing standard, and this is perceived as an important element in Latvia's efforts to act on the social determinants of health and reduce inequities in health *(47)*.

To increase capacity, the districts were abolished and 109 municipalities and 9 republican cities were created in July 2009 *(48)*. As these changes were implemented recently, the effects on local government capacity and tackling inequities in health and social determinants remain unknown.

Despite the decentralization process, the significance in Latvia of national (and EU) policy frameworks prescribing and often guaranteeing social services such as good housing, education, health care and a minimum income should not be underestimated. Our respondent argued that, for Latvia, this was essential in tackling inequities in health and the social determinants of health, and the financial support to do is also indispensable.

At the central level, the Ministry of Welfare has committed to reducing inequities in health and accepted a quantitative target of a 25% reduction (measured by using multiple indicators) by 2010. Latvia's economy is currently performing poorly (unemployment above the EU average and national income significantly lower than the EU average) following the international economic crisis. In general, the person interviewed suggested that local politicians give local plans the necessary political backbone by supporting proposed programmes that give more detail on how they want to tackle inequities in health and the social determinants of health and contribute to achieving the national target.

Other key stakeholders for local government action on social determinants of health and inequities in health that were identified during the interview include the Ministry of Health, the Latvian Association of Municipalities and the Latvian Large Cities Association. For municipalities, the importance of creating, supporting and increasing local capacity was also identified: "It is very important to give support to [civil] society activities, which can be done in many different ways. It could be an office for a nongovernmental organization or by including different groups in the policy-making process." In turn, nongovernmental organizations were recognized to be an important link between the municipality and deprived groups. "Nongovernmental organizations are important in a social context. Besides, they communicate social needs to the municipality."

3.3.3.3 Netherlands

The Netherlands has a subnational tier of government – the provinces – between the municipal and national governments. The provinces are responsible for spatial planning, transport and, together with municipalities, financing and regulating services for young people. Nationally, the Social Support Act and the Public Health Act are the key pieces of legislation for improving access to health care and reducing inequities in health. The Social Support Act covers nine domains,[3] each with its own target groups and goals. The responsibilities stipulated by the Social Support Act come with a defined budget for some domains but not for improving social welfare. However, the municipalities have relatively high autonomy to decide how to achieve the goals of the Social Support Act. Improving the social determinants of health and inequities in health are hot political topics but are also considered a policy area in which little successful progress has been made politically or at the policy level. Fiscal pressure from providing social care to older people was cited as a growing problem for municipalities.

At the municipal level, a local politician has explicit responsibility for complying with the Social Support Act, but this was not considered to always make implementation more successful, possibly because, despite the local politician having responsibility, there was thought to be little real accountability for successful delivery. Local government often cooperates with the local municipal health service, which covers several municipalities and is jointly owned by local governments. The municipal health service provides a range

---

[3] Promoting social cohesion; prevention targeted at youth/young adults and parents with parenting problems; providing citizens with info; support carers and volunteers; stimulating social involvement and independent functioning of the disabled or people with psychosocial problems; providing social services for the disabled or people with psychosocial problems ; providing social care (including care for women); promoting public health; promoting addiction policy.

of public health services, including mapping inequities in health.

3.3.3.4 Spain

In Spain, two national laws, the federal health law and the cohesion law for the National Health Service, refer to the social determinants of health. However, regional government is very important within Spain. The autonomous communities have substantial independence from the central government, with virtually all responsibility for health devolved to the autonomous communities. The levels of governance are coordinated through formal and informal mechanisms. Nationally, there are formal coordination bodies across the autonomous communities and national government. Autonomous communities also work with non-health departments, including education, economics and social services to address inequities in health and the social determinants of health, although the interviewee suggested that this work is perceived to have varying success.

At the level of the autonomous communities focused on here, the interviewee said that tackling social determinants of health and inequities in health is on the political agenda but as a relatively recent phenomenon. The interviewee perceived that the term "social determinants of health" was not often used at the national level. Within Aragon, regional government health law refers to tackling inequities in health through the social determinants of health, and a further draft law is being developed that aims to make tackling these determinants central to all health policies. Work on this topic is funded through general revenue except for specific programmes related to vulnerable communities such as people living with HIV.

Several other autonomous communities were considered active in tackling inequities in health: Andalucía, Catalonia and Valencia. However, the pattern of action and the division of action between the autonomous community and the municipal governments varied across those autonomous communities. In Aragon, the municipalities (except for Zaragoza) are small, and the municipalities therefore have limited capacity to focus on inequities in health and the social determinants of health. Municipalities in rural areas often have relatively small budgets, which provides little financial or staff capacity or flexibility for separate action to tackle inequities in health. The interviewee perceived that the level of political commitment across the autonomous communities and the municipalities varies, mainly because of a lack of recognition of the issue rather than a lack of concern for the population.

3.3.3.5 Sweden

In Sweden, action to tackle the social determinants of health and inequities in health is on the agenda at both the national and local levels. The 21 county councils are responsible for purchasing and providing health care at the regional level, are largely autonomous of the state and collect taxes. The county councils and 290 municipalities share responsibility for the broader agenda on the social determinants of health. Municipalities are responsibility for the social welfare agenda and are again largely autonomous of the county councils and the national government. General budgets embed funding to tackle social determinants of health and inequities in health, and there is no separately identified budget unless a county council or municipality allocates specific funding.

The interviewee said that action to tackle the social determinants of health and inequities in health is embedded within the broader system across the national, regional and local levels, both at the policy and fiscal level. The report of the Commission on Social Determinants of Health *(1)* was specifically cited as instrumental in opening the policy window in Sweden. The perception was that the role of social determinants in improving health and reducing inequities in health was a significant political aspiration. The respondent also emphasized that politicians from both the right and the left were committed to reducing inequities in health, although from different perspectives, with the right focusing on the right to access to health care and the left focusing on equality and equity. Despite these differences in focus, politicians locally sought to agree on ways to tackle the agenda.

3.3.4 Summary of emerging themes

The interviews with local authorities on structure, governance and fiscal context revealed several important themes for the social determinants of health and inequities in health. Four are especially important: differences in governance structures and capacity levels, expenditure levels and identifying funding, the wider legislative framework and accountability.

3.3.4.1 Differences in governance structures and capacity levels

Countries in the European Region differ significantly in subnational governance structures. This may seem self-evident, but the differences, complexities and the vastly different structures and levels of power need to be explicitly acknowledged. The local authorities interviewed here include powerful regions such as Aragon and Västra Götaland County Council, which have the power to raise taxes and have significant opportunity to set their own policy context.

By contrast, the local authorities interviewed in Denmark and the Netherlands had less power, less ability to collect taxes and less influence over their policy context than other respondents. In some instances, the legal and financial context is even significantly different across tiers that have similar names and appear to operate at similar levels within the wider system, such as the differences in role and scope of control between municipalities in Spain and the Netherlands, despite their apparently similar position in the system. All these factors strongly influence the autonomy with which various forms of local government can act on the social determinants of health. Interviewees from countries in which the regions have tax-collecting powers described considerable autonomy from the national government. However, in Spain and Sweden, this independence was mirrored by the independence of the municipalities from the regions. This heterogeneity leads to very different capacity to build strong programmes of action to tackle the social determinants of health and inequities in health across systems and countries.

3.3.4.2 Expenditure levels and identifying funding

Expenditure levels, and especially the ability to define the budget for social determinants of health, comprised a common theme across every interview. Almost every interviewee observed that, although identifying money that is labelled and given to specific programmes is relatively simple, defining the total budget spent on improving the social determinants of health and inequities in health is difficult. A particular difficulty was the need to include a variety of closely linked policy areas, such as education, public transport, public safety and the department in charge of spatial planning.

3.3.4.3 The wider legislative framework

The wider legislative framework around local government is critical for action on the social determinants of health and inequities in health. In many of the interviewees' countries, tackling inequities in health is part of governments' larger responsibility for the well-being of their citizens but is marked by vague and unfunded commitments. Several interviewees emphasized that legislation often includes such terms as health promotion and well-being for all, but commitments or quantification to bridge the gradient are seldom made *(49)*. The literature also reflects this, with Judge et al. *(50)* differentiating three groups of countries: two in which targets are generally set (including England and the Netherlands) and one group

– the Czech Republic, Latvia and Lithuania – following recommendations made by the World Bank. Second, beyond the general legislative framework, several municipalities said that some social determinants of health have their own field of legislation, such as safety in the workplace. When this is the case, legislation and strategic papers more often set targets for tackling the problem. Legislation directly linked to inequities in health or the social determinants of health often remains vague, whereas specific legislation linked to one of the determinants of health is often more clear.

The types of interventions differed significantly across the local authorities interviewed. In particular, the local authorities in central and eastern Europe appeared to have a larger role in providing social services and tackling poverty. However, this also means that reducing inequities in health largely depends on the national economic situation. The municipality in Latvia was very concerned about the effects of the economic downturn. The municipalities' range of social services and programmes is expected to decrease, and pending unemployment and predicted increasing poverty will increase the demand for social benefits and are likely to increase inequities in health. The interviewee from Latvia therefore said that, considering the economic downturn, "not losing our successes will be the biggest challenge for the future".

3.3.4.4 Accountability

The governance and legislative context also raised important questions on accountability within local government. Only one interviewee – from the Netherlands – said that someone in local government is directly responsible for tackling the social determinants of health and inequities in health. In this case, it was a member of the executive board responsible for social determinants of health through the Social Support Act. It is debatable whether having accountability at the executive level is a wise investment: the interviewee from the local authority in the Netherlands doubted whether this accountability benefited the actual implementation. However, other interviewees were seriously concerned that accountability would be an important potential lever for change. Another interviewee said that making everybody responsible for the social determinants of health and reducing inequities in health meant that no one would be responsible. As another interviewee said, "sometimes action is so embedded in the system that it is hard to see it". The lack of accountability at the executive level in some local authorities and the doubts of its efficacy therefore raise important questions for debate as local authorities seek to work effectively on the social determinants of health.

3.4 Action on tackling the social determinants of health

All the authorities interviewed have programmes in place to address inequities in health through the social determinants of health, although the programmes differ in scope, focus and content.

Four areas for action identified in the report of the Commission on Social Determinants of Health were selected for particular investigation through the interviews with the local authorities. The aim was to link local governments' initiatives with the objectives set out in the report. Areas were selected to reflect their importance in tackling inequities in health and to show the wider role of local government. The interviewees were therefore asked to describe activity to tackle inequities in health and social determinants of health for the following groups or areas:

- children and young people;
- fighting poverty and unemployment;
- creating and developing healthy and sustainable places and communities; and
- older people.

The following section describes their range of activities. Nevertheless, this is not intended to be an exhaustive list of programmes and activities.

3.4.1 Children and young people

Action on tackling inequities in health in relation to children and young people was high on the agenda, with all interviewees considering early intervention as a priority. The topics addressed included drug and alcohol abuse, promotion of physical activity and promotion of safe sex. This approach may suggest that an approach oriented towards lifestyles was adopted rather than a focus on the social determinants of health across the social gradient.

The Aragon region has several funding programmes designed to support and promote locally based action. Some of their programmes required intersectoral working and innovation, with more than 60 local initiatives being funded this way. They have also established a fund for schools. "Access to the school fund requires a programme of work taking place for a minimum of three years on five key topics: diet, physical fitness, drugs and alcohol, environment and mental health. This work is also specifically aimed at reducing inequities in health, with a focus on the most vulnerable students and their parents and families." Other programmes targeted the most vulnerable members of society, including HIV prevention with sex workers. Nongovernmental organizations and other social partners carried out much of the work directly, but the Autonomous Community funded it.

Denmark provides an even more individual focus by having health or social workers create health profiles of children. "When children leave ninth grade, a doctor or nurse examines them and health profiles are individually created. If the profile that emerges is negative, social and health care workers try to react." This enables inequities in health to be mapped and monitored.

In Jurmula, Latvia, an annual Family Sports Day is organized to promote physical activity. "We [also] stimulate safe behaviour on the streets and show the effects of drug and alcohol abuse." Alcohol abuse is drawn into a larger context in Maastricht, Netherlands by including the family: "We have a programme that targets families and shows the consequences of alcohol abuse for their relational environment."

Another example of a programme came from Maastricht, with a school programme aimed at promoting awareness of the importance of healthy living and good nutrition. In Sweden, the interviewee has also been working together with the Ministry of Education and Research to promote focusing on health values and health education when teaching.

All interviewees considered work with children and young people to be an important investment for the future and identified it as the area that needed the most attention. This theme also illustrated both the scale and breadth of work taking place at the subnational level. Nevertheless, action through mainstream budgets such as housing and transport was less frequent, although some interviewees stressed the importance of education to stimulate social mobility.

3.4.2 Fighting poverty and unemployment

Many of the initiatives the interviewees highlighted in this area focused on workplace health. In Denmark, each employer addresses the effects of the working environment on the health and well-being of workers through a workplace audit. Each employer has to undertake a full audit of the workplace to assess the health effects on workers. The audit has to address effects on physical and mental health and monitor progress on any problems. All employers conduct a full audit every three years.

In Sweden, policies in relation to the work and employment agenda are perceived as being largely reactive, although interest is growing on the health effects of work-related stress. This was particularly in relation to the sense of control for workers and the level of demands being put on individuals. The Netherlands had several initiatives focusing on promoting a safe and healthy working environment, especially work–life balance.

In Latvia, some municipalities provide social benefits to unemployed people, supported by the European Social Fund. Municipalities also have a statutory responsibility to provide housing and minimum income levels for their inhabitants. This is supplemented by other financial benefits for the citizens with the lowest incomes, including school meals, childcare and funding for necessities for school free of charge. However, the economic crisis is biting deeply in Latvia: municipal budgets are being cut and they are losing staff. This makes planning for more work on the social determinants of health and inequities in health very difficult.

3.4.3 Creating and developing healthy and sustainable places and communities

Interest is growing in creating and developing healthy and sustainable places. All interviewees mentioned a wide range of projects, including promoting physical activity, such as walking and cycling, and using inequities in health as a lever for improving air quality.

The promotion of physical activity appears to be popular in all municipalities, although many interviewees expressed concern that this risks increasing inequities in health. One interviewee said: "To a great extent physical activity is picked up by the middle and upper class and, to a lesser extent, disadvantaged groups." Another approach to introducing physical activity was the financial promotion of bicycles among social and health care workers in Aarhus, Denmark. "We have a pilot project introducing bicycles to care workers, who often have lower income. The care workers are quite keen to use these bicycles."

A range of other work linked to air quality and environmental degradation was reported, including action to reduce airborne particulate matter by using tunnels for major roads and urban development programmes to reduce segregation. "In this case, proven regional inequities in health appeared to be a lever for developing a tunnel aiming to reduce the intensity of the particulate. This proved that the social determinants of health do influence the agenda on urban governance." However, municipalities reported that getting inequities in health and the social determinants of health structurally included in the built environment agenda is often a difficult process. Of the local authorities interviewed, the ones in Sweden and Denmark were alone in reporting that discussion of the built environment as a key determinant for health has been growing within the region.

In Maastricht, the interviewee felt that "there is room for improvement in various areas, such as spatial planning. When (urban) plans are developed, health is one of the topics taken into account but not the most important topic." Jurmula has also made an effort to include tackling social determinants of health and inequities in health: "Health is a very important aspect in the Development Strategy for 2010–2016. It sets out what the municipality has to realize in the field of health in a broad sense, considering all determinants of health: housing and the cultural and social environment."

3.4.4 Older people

All the interviewees recognized older people as a target group in tackling the social determinants of health and inequities in health. In particular, numerous public services appear to be very important for older people. The interviewee from the Netherlands noted: "Access to public transport for older people – and vulnerable groups in general – is very important. If they do not have good access to local and regional public transport, they need individual tools to participate in society and to avoid the risk of social deprivation." The Municipality of Jurmula also promotes public transport to sustain an active old age.

Many more activities are aimed at including older people and promoting an active lifestyle. In Aragon, "The department of social services has now started a programme in which they encourage older people to travel abroad for a reduced price." The department of culture in Jurmula "supports cultural activities for all ages, including dancing groups and choirs for middle-aged people and seniors". However, access to social services remains the main concern of municipalities. "As with all target groups ... you need to bring services to people so, for instance, we provide services within nursing homes."

3.4.5 Summary

These examples illustrate the wide breadth of action possible for local government. These demonstrate the following.

- Local government is pursuing the agenda on improving health and tackling inequities in health, specifically through the social determinants of health.
- Action is being developed across not only the key areas set out in the Commission on Social Determinants of Health report but also more broadly, bringing in a wide range of local government responsibilities and nuanced into the specific culture and legal framework of the country or region.
- Local civic, political and executive leadership is important in orchestrating partnerships based on a whole-system approach supported by organizational development programmes to empower citizens in a more asset-based approach to building social capital.

However, the examples also demonstrate gaps in this activity.

- Health was rarely a key focus for action in spatial planning and the built environment. Some interviewees considered this a source of frustration: "… this is odd, as urban governance is often linked to social improvement while social improvement is constrained by inequities in health." The WHO European Healthy Cities Network also recognizes the lack of (qualitative) environmental initiatives, and commentators have suggested that barriers between actors and the difficulty of integrating programmes are important factors *(51)*.
- There were also clear gaps in activities aiming to work across the gradient rather than targeting specific groups despite the clear evidence showing that national, regional and local government working in partnership with all key agencies needs to take action across the social gradient on the social determinants of health in a concerted effort. If inequities in health occur as a consequence of social inequality, then several agencies and individuals with cross-cutting policies and a focus on equity in health need to take action. A lack of understanding, appreciation and acknowledgement of the social determinants of health means that programmes and projects frequently target the most disadvantaged people at the bottom of the social gradient in health. Even when some of these are effective, they fail to tackle the inequities across other socioeconomic groups across the social gradient. Scaled up and systematic action is required that is universal but proportionate to the disadvantage across the social gradient. This is a prerequisite for effective delivery to addressing inequities in health.

Both of these areas raise important questions on the understanding of the social determinants of health, the capacity within local government and how to translate political willingness into practical action.

3.5 Implementing action on the social determinants of health

Although the political and fiscal context of local government and the ongoing initiatives of local authorities in the European Region are both important, the question of how to practically implement change is also key to action on the social determinants of health and inequities in health. However, the existing literature on implementing action to tackle the social determinants of health and inequities in health is relatively weak. The interviews therefore especially emphasized exploring implementation and the experience of local government in attempting to carry out constructive change.

All the local authorities interviewed had addressing inequities in health and the social determinants of health firmly on their agendas: clearly tackling the social determinants of health and inequities in health is becoming a priority in local government at both the political and staff levels. However, exploring how this is being translated into practice is important: is it mainly rhetoric, or are politicians really dedicated to tackling the problem? Are countries showing concern, do they have a will to take action or are they really undertaking action *(52)*? As the previous section highlighted, certain social determinants of health tend to receive more focus than others. In addition, the interviewees highlighted numerous implementation issues, even in the areas in which more work on tackling inequities in health was taking place. Although some of these factors were country-specific, many were common themes across all the local authorities interviewed.

Six key implementation factors were highlighted: the level of intersectoral cooperation, policy coherence, the strength and communication of the evidence base, capacity, managing the political context and knowledge transfer.

3.5.1 Intersectoral cooperation
All the interviewees highlighted the need for action on the agenda on the social determinants of health and inequities in health to be taken across organizational, sectoral and geographical boundaries. The interviewees frequently expressed the need for this as a need to maximize impact and minimize effort, and many municipalities expressed anxiety that the difficulties and resource implications of working across multiple boundaries led to poorly coordinated action that risked contradicting or duplicating core objectives: "Too often we see that similar programmes are duplicated across different areas and over different disciplines."

Most of the interviewees have a mix of formal and informal structures in place to address this. However, the breadth of the agenda on the social determinants of health and inequities in health and the need for broad-based intersectoral action in most countries has led to complex partnership arrangements for many of the local authorities interviewed. Although including multiple stakeholders is commonly agreed to be important, the complexity of multiple agendas and perspectives makes reaching consensus difficult. As one interviewee said: "A clear agreement on target groups and efficient solutions would contribute to better tackling of inequities in health." Although the interviewees therefore accept a central role of local government in tackling inequities in health, a clearly identified implementation challenge is building and strengthening the leadership role of local government, especially working across sectors coordinating initiatives.

3.5.2 Policy coherence and incoherence
All interviewees consider the local aspect of the work of local government to be important in meeting the needs of specific communities. Nevertheless, the proliferation of local action means that many of the interviewees found that evaluation has become difficult to carry out and policy coherence difficult to achieve. Coherence can be defined as consistency of policy objectives free from self-contradiction, in which action for implementation does not undermine policies and adverse consequences are avoided. This becomes more difficult when operating in partnership within a complex, adaptive system to address the social determinants of health in which outcomes are unpredictable and unintended *(53)*. In the words of one interviewee: "There is a common interest [in social determinants], and everybody is committed to the overarching goal, but decision-making remains very difficult because

there are too many options." This is considered a problem, as ensuring that action is focused for maximum impact could become difficult. Assessing impact also requires a high level of understanding and monitoring of the local actions, both for wider dissemination if something is seen to be working but also to determine whether a change in focus is needed if something is not delivering the expected outcome. The search for coherence therefore raises important questions, in particular about the effectiveness of scaling up small interventions and how locally based interventions can be transferred into different contexts.

Although the interviewees acknowledged the leadership role of local government in bringing together key stakeholders, all the municipalities covered highlighted the difficulty of bringing policy coherence at a national level to a wide range of small, often very locally based initiatives. In the words of one interviewee: "It is important to translate those small and effective practices to a more national and international level." Some interviewees raised the need for greater policy coherence between the different tiers of government: national, regional and local. To enforce policy coherence, some countries (Denmark, the Netherlands and Sweden) have national programmes or targets. However, these targets often refer to a target group (such as children) or a social determinant of health (such as the physical environment or working conditions). The success of this approach is unclear. What is clear is that the positive alignment of policy at all levels is considered critical in achieving the synergy and impact needed to address inequities in health and shift the steepness of the social gradient *(1)*. For local government, this can be considered at two levels. First, there is the task of achieving coherence of policy-making at the national, regional and local levels. Alongside this is achieving strategic fit and coherence between local strategic plans and objectives involving partner agencies and the role and remit of discrete projects to deliver these objectives *(54)*.

3.5.3 Evidence base

Most interviewees raised a common implementation issue: the lack of a substantial evidence base on what works that local government could use. The interviews suggest that many local governments seem to have achieved a level of political commitment, albeit at varying levels.

However, one interviewee highlighted the need to be able to follow up with a clear evidence-informed plan that was appropriate to the local context: "... policy has to be scientifically underpinned".

In the view of the interviewees, the lack of evidence on interventions is manifested in both a lack of available evidence to inform the current and future work and also the difficulty of evaluating the programmes already in place.

This is a particular issue in terms of bending mainstream budgets such as those for housing, education and transport to the agenda of improving health and reducing inequities in health. Interviewees commonly requested more sharing of learning on measuring social determinants of health and inequities in health and learning on how to effectively implement programmes to tackle them. The two regional governments interviewed saw part of their role as facilitating knowledge sharing across municipalities and between regions.

Most interviewees argued that any evidence base needed to include not only examples of effective work elsewhere but also sufficient information to allow authorities to focus their efforts and, as far as possible, to scope any additional capacity needed. Encouragingly, however, none of the authorities interviewed viewed the lack of evidence as a reason not to take action. However, all the authorities expressed concern that they were having to navigate in the dark with little evidence for their activity, often little capacity to evaluate what they were doing and having to extrapolate from evidence from various sectors to guide their action. The interviewees recognized that a full-fledged evidence base was not available but repeated their desire that the available evidence be collected and be disseminated.

3.5.4 Capacity

The interviews also revealed significant differences in the capacity of local government to take action on the social determinants of health and inequities in health. These capacity issues concerned in particular the internal organizational capacity of some municipalities serving small populations, which also face very limited flexibility in planning and delivering services due to the wider policy and legislative context. Despite their size, the smaller local authorities interviewed felt a strong need to have a voice in the discussion at the national and international levels.

The interviews also revealed gaps in understanding certain aspects of the social determinants of health and inequities in health. For example, although all interviewees discussed initiatives attempting to use the social determinants of health to tackle inequities in health, few discussed the difference between targeting vulnerable groups and working across the whole gradient. Most interviewees were seeking solutions through very focused work, such as targeting small geographical areas and specific communities to focus interventions on the most vulnerable communities. The interviews therefore suggest that the discussion on targeting versus working across the gradient is therefore an important area of capacity development in local government and one that will materially affect implementation. Without a clear understanding of the cause of the causes of inequities in health, action is likely to be ineffective, project-driven and inappropriately targeted at the bottom of the social gradient. Proportionate universal policies and action focused across the life course on the social determinants of health require clarity of understanding, strategy and concerted leadership across the key agencies to be effective.

3.5.5 Managing the political context

All interviewees highlighted the importance of political commitment for this agenda and reported increased political commitment. The strength of the political commitment ranged from clear leadership (either at the national or local level) through to political permission to pursue the agenda. Much work has clearly been underway to get the social determinants of health and inequities in health onto the political agenda, and this work appears to have been successful, at least in part. Several interviewees mentioned the strength of political leadership as a factor in the success of developing the agenda, although several also raised the need for greater political leadership.

Although all interviewees expressed a desire to understand the actions that are being taken elsewhere, they did not specifically mention understanding the arguments used to get the social determinants of health and inequities in health on the agenda. However, there is a clear opportunity to learn from the countries that have been successful in increasing political commitment. The interviewees felt that identifying a common approach or set of factors that might be developed and adapted for use in a variety of settings could potentially support the rapid development of this agenda within local government. The central role of political leadership in this agenda must therefore not be overlooked in developing tools to support local government in this work.

3.5.6 Knowledge transfer

All interviewees were keen to understand the actions and outcomes from other places and to be able to transfer knowledge into their own situation. One interviewee argued: "Especially within the area of evaluating implemented programmes, sometimes it is difficult to evaluate the exact impact of certain programmes on reducing inequities in health." Another interviewee experienced difficulty in working intersectorally and would therefore like to know how to implement intersectoral strategies. Yet another interviewee said: "The added value would be in sharing knowledge, but I would also like to see more collaboration between regions on concrete topics: for example, measurement issues, methodology, initiatives or programmes." There seems to be a strong and often underused opportunity for international learning and exchange. This is not to underestimate the potential complexity of transferring knowledge across the different local government contexts: transferring learning in a country between similar tiers of government might be relatively straightforward, but the substantial differences in settings require a very nuanced approach to knowledge transfer. Despite differences in political climate, financing mechanisms and system culture, the challenges local government faces often resonate across many countries.

3.5.7 Summary of the interview outcomes

The interviews clearly showed that, in general, local authorities are committed to the principle of working on the social determinants of health and inequities in health. The engagement of politicians and political leadership is developing at the local and regional levels. However, after they get inequities in health onto the political agenda, many local authorities face the challenge of keeping it there, developing the understanding and involvement across local government and overcoming the significant challenges of implementation. The interviews suggest that the lessons from this success in the work to put inequities in health and the social determinants of health on the agenda could be usefully analysed and captured but that the key challenge now is to build evidence and capacity to implement change effectively and sustainably.

3.6 Policy implications of the interviews with local authorities

The interviews with local authorities, especially on the reality of practical implementation, suggest several important considerations for taking forward the agenda of the social determinants of health in local government.

3.6.1 Understanding the differences between local government contexts

In the small sample from this study, the local government contexts ranged from highly autonomous regional governments with tax-raising powers to small municipalities with highly dispersed populations, small budgets and limited revenue-raising powers. Activity to support implementation in local government or to build the evidence base needs to take account of these significant differences and to be able to be nuanced in the various political and organizational settings.

These local authorities clearly strongly desire to learn from what is working well. Nevertheless, the diversity and complexity of the structural and legal frameworks for local government across the European Region means that a one-size-fits-all approach to transferring international learning will fail. A nuanced approach that makes explicit not just the content of interventions but also the implicit competencies might better support the rapid spread of learning.

3.6.2 Building political commitment

All the interviewees highlighted the importance of political commitment for producing action within local government. The interviewees especially highlighted the importance of getting and maintaining political commitment in relation both to the leadership role of local government and the allocation of funding. In the words of one interviewee: "More funds are needed for health promotion and disease prevention; too much money is spent on improving health services and hospitals." In developing tools to support taking forward this agenda within local government, the central importance of local political leadership should therefore be explicitly recognized and supported.

3.6.3 Transferring knowledge

Local governments across the European Region are at very different stages in tackling the agenda of social determinants of health and inequities in health. Although all the local authorities interviewed had social determinants of health and inequities in health on the agenda, action to support local government in acting on political willingness needs to be put in place rapidly. Learning from other countries and those that have already taken action can be usefully shared. The local authorities interviewed specifically requested this, especially those still too small to command a strong voice in national and international discussions.

3.6.4 Building capacity for action on inequities in health and the social determinants of health

The understanding of the role of local government and the potential range of actions available appears to be more developed in themes more commonly associated with inequities in health such as services for and prevention work with children and young people and work with vulnerable communities. Relatively little evidence indicates that this agenda has significantly penetrated into more mainstream local government work such as urban development or antipoverty work. In transport, the focus appears to be mainly on encouraging and facilitating walking and cycling. The rhetoric of "bending mainstream budgets to tackle inequities in health" does not seem to be blocked by lack of political commitment but by a lack of understanding and evidence of what that might actually mean in practice. Practical examples of how authorities have managed to build action on social determinants into mainstream agendas are needed.

3.6.5 Cooperation and partnership

The interviews indicated that municipalities are most active in addressing issues for children and young people whereas areas such as spatial planning sometimes lagged behind. Several municipalities indicated that they see a more important role for urban governance in tackling inequities in health but that they were struggling to get social determinants of health and inequities in health onto the spatial planning agenda.

Why do programmes aimed at children and young people and at young adults appear to be more widespread? One explanation the local authorities offered is that the well-being of one group (such as children and young people or young adults) assembles actors with one common goal, improving the lives of children and young people, making cooperation easier. However, in spatial planning and urban development, actors have divergent interests, and health and well-being are rarely the key drivers. To stimulate addressing the social determinants of health, "adequate inclusive and empowering policy responses should be directed at combating the polarising mechanisms in central arenas such as the labour market, the housing market, social services and education" *(55)*.

This has been recognized since the early 1990s and is the reason that Denmark and the Netherlands, for instance, introduced models in which social housing agencies, schools, municipalities and local entrepreneurs work together to improve deprived neighbourhoods. Whether this approach is successful has yet to be determined. Some commentators criticize the approach for relocating deprived neighbourhoods within cities.

3.6.6 Building policy and legislative structures and frameworks that enable action

All the interviewees highlighted the importance of the political and fiscal structures in which local authorities are embedded for influencing the opportunities for tackling inequities in health and the social determinants of health.

Structures need to be enabling: municipalities need a legal basis for carrying out tasks. One example for which enabling instruments and structures are particularly important is the question of coordination.

Partnership is inherent to successfully tackling inequities in health, as many social determinants of health have a major non-health aspect. Many interviewees acknowledged that multiple departments or actors are often working on the same subject, almost working in the same way, but are still not cooperating. Several interviewees suggested the value of supportive instruments for coordination: legal, fiscal or both. The Social Support Act in the Netherlands is a useful example, although some fine-tuning is still needed. Programmes that bring together multiple parties and channel the funding stream were also highlighted (Spain).

4. Final conclusions and implications for the WHO European Healthy Cities Network

The report of the Commission on Social Determinants of Health and the subsequent strategic review of health inequalities in England post-2010 have provided a robust framework and evidence for action emphasizing the link between social conditions, social inequalities, inequities in health and health status. Globally, the Commission on Social Determinants of Health recommended improving the material conditions within which people are born, learn, live, work and age and the distribution of psychosocial well-being within neighbourhoods and communities that are socially cohesive and where people can exercise control over their lives. This firmly places equity in health at the heart of urban governance and planning.

Fair society, healthy lives (26) gathered the best global and national evidence together in relation to inequalities in health to identify the interventions most likely to be effective in England. It reinforced social justice as the key driver requiring concerted action on inequities in health across the whole population. The economic, psychosocial and environmental context of people's lifelong experience influence and constrain lifestyle choices. *Fair society, healthy lives (26)* identified the need to focus on the social determinants of health – early years, education and training, social protection, decent work, economic status and income and access to resources and services, including but not restricted to health care, housing and transport that facilitate personal control and participation in healthy and flourishing neighbourhoods and communities.

The key principles that apply to healthy cities include the following.

- Social justice, health and sustainability should be at the heart of all policies nationally, regionally and locally to create a common value base for concerted partnership action.
- Improving health and well-being and reducing inequities in health require empowering individuals and communities to take control, promoting personal well-being, community participation, social cohesion and equity. People, process and place are key dimensions.
- The public sector should provide new forms of political, civic and public leadership focused on creating the conditions within which people and communities can take control of their lives.
- Strategies intervening in just one part of the system are generally insufficient to make the necessary difference or affect only a minority of the population. Action is required on the social determinants of health across the whole population proportionally to the level of disadvantage and across the life course to address the cumulative effect of inequities in health.
- Strategies and policies need to be crosscutting at the national, regional and local levels. Inequity in health has multiple causes, is multidimensional and complex and requires action at all levels in a range of agencies and sectors. This requires sophisticated partnership working across complex organizational and sector boundaries.
- Experience so far suggests that broad principles for action can be developed, but solutions are not straightforward across disparate regions, cities, towns and villages, and solutions need be tailored to specific cultural, historical and geographical contexts (framework for action *(6)*: sections 4.1.2, 4.3, 5.1, 5.3.1 and 5.4).

The review argued for a wide role for local government in England in addressing inequalities. Key roles identified for local government include:

- providing community leadership to extend civic participation and local governance, mobilizing communities to co-produce health and well-being and to develop social capital, trust and resilience;
- identifying individual and population needs and assets to inform strategic approaches and partnership working in taking local action on the social determinants of inequalities in health;
- promoting safe and sustainable places and communities, undertaking health equity impact assessment in urban planning and place shaping to inform new design and the regeneration of existing neighbourhoods;
- commissioning and providing a range of direct and evidence-informed prevention services to engage individuals and neighbourhoods consistent with statutory duties;
- regulating consistent with devolved local powers to address inequalities in health; and
- where local government is a major employer, directly or indirectly using commissioning, contracting and the provision of employment to improve local employment conditions (framework for action *(6)*: sections 4.1, 4.3, 5.5 and 5.8.2).

4.1 The role of local government: a view across six countries

The report considers the approaches of local government to inequities in health across six countries: Denmark, England, Latvia, the Netherlands, Spain and Sweden. This enables consideration of models of strong national, regional and municipal leadership.

The analysis emphasizes that local government does not represent one single entity but is complex and disparate, with different structures, political and financial arrangement and levels of power. More powerful players raise taxes and set their own policy agendas, whereas others are not empowered to do so. Acknowledging these differences in structures, roles and autonomy reveals differences in the capacity to scale up the activity needed to address the social determinants of health. Understanding this and the wider legislative framework within which regions and municipalities operate is a prerequisite for understanding the role of local government.

The types of intervention at various levels of government differ substantially. Nevertheless, evidence indicates that local governments are taking a broad range of initiatives focused on inequities in health and the social determinants of health. This clearly demonstrates the commitment of local governments to play a significant role in responding to the needs of their local population, however they are defined. Within this positive stance, several gaps are identified that need to be explored further. These relate particularly to action on equity in health through work and the use of activity around place to understand and reduce inequities in health. This has been recognized in the interviews undertaken for this review and by the WHO Healthy Cities movement.

Place shaping in cities is a significant role for local government in improving health. People need good places to live if they are to enjoy good health and well-being. These are characterized by good services, availability of high-quality housing, access to employment and a sense of safety and community, leading to high levels of social capital and personal and collective psychosocial well-being. The communities in which people live significantly influence their health and mental well-being. Place and the social networks to which people belong across their life course have telling effects on their health.

However, the social, economic and environmental resources that drive such well-being are not equally distributed. Using equity and well-being lenses potentially extends the scope for implementing social determinants models of health and well-being.

In this model, local government becomes identified not solely as a provider of services but as supporting a better life for its citizens, nurturing psychosocial well-being at both the individual and population levels. This focus, when placed within an asset-based approach, builds social capital and community resources rather than describing deficits, problems and needs.

Such upstream activity may well make economic sense in a time of recession, when local authorities are likely to retrench to core services and communities face challenges to well-being through increased unemployment, debt and threats to social cohesion. Increasing individual and collective resilience through early action on health and psychosocial well-being may well produce a significant response.

Much of the evidence base for the social determinants of health has been known for some time, although it is currently more robust and better collated. The evidence on implementation and delivery is less developed.

This report has identified six implementation factors of particular importance:
- multiagency, multidisciplinary partnerships and collaboration;
- policy alignment and convergence;
- the robustness of the evidence base;
- developing capability and capacity;
- managing the political environment; and
- transferring knowledge.

4.2 Multiagency and multidisciplinary partnership and collaboration

Partnership working is identified as a key prerequisite in taking action on the social determinants of health, because this requires comprehensive action by a range of stakeholders working in a concerted and sustained way to address the issues. Significant barriers can be identified to developing mature partnership working. These include lack of understanding of the key drivers of the social determinants of health and artificially separating health policy from other relevant policies, leading to displacement of responsibility. The latter can be compounded by the inability to separately identify the total money spent on the social determinants of health. This appears to be a common feature across all the countries and needs to be systematically addressed. Overall, although partnership working is generally a feature, little systematic evaluation has established whether such partnerships deliver better health outcomes. There are, however, some pointers to developing mature partnerships capable of delivery. A key requirement for effective partnerships is a new and different model of leadership focused on a whole-system approach and grounded in the active participation of communities. It needs to be based on co-production of health and well-being in a delivery model that shifts the balance of power towards local people and communities and away from professionals and formal institutions. Evidence from implementation suggests that the above approach frees up local policy-makers, citizens and communities to tailor specific solutions to local problems – with more explicit local accountability – when it is linked with clarity of strategic direction between agencies and explicit agreement on joint priorities, with targets limited to those necessary to drive strategic goals. Achieving the synergy needed to sustain progress requires coherence of strategy, policy and delivery across the whole system consistent with the values and principles of social justice *(56)*. Partnership structures, formal and informal, are a part of the total picture, and these need to be refined to maximize their effects in facilitating delivery (framework for action *(6)*: sections 4.1, 5.2, 5.5 and 5.8.6).

4.3 Policy alignment and convergence

The need for coherence between policies at the various level of government is critical. Alignment at all levels is critically important to secure coherence of approach between strategy at various levels and local delivery *(56)*. Unless this can be secured, the synergy necessary to scale up from local initiatives into national objectives becomes obscured and promotes drift back into small-scale initiatives focused on lifestyles and behaviour change. The tensions in partnership working in securing agreed and explicit priorities have been well documented, and these reinforce the earlier commentary on the new forms of leadership across the public sector, which can take a whole-system approach and embrace models of dispersed leadership that engage citizens, communities and organizations at all levels (framework for action *(6)*: sections 4.1, 4.3, 5.1, 5.5 and 6.3).

4.4 The robustness of the evidence base
There is a general view that, although the evidence base on the social determinants of health has strengthened during the past decade, the evidence base on what works remains relatively weak. Each country can produce evidence of best practices, but this has not yet been collated, although some documents attempt to bring together various initiatives and evaluate the national programme. More dynamic processes for sharing best practices are developing, but the knowledge base of what works needs to be strengthened and good practices disseminated effectively nationally and internationally. This requires more systematically evaluating activity on the social determinants of health and creating structures capable of ensuring effective dissemination across all the key stakeholders (framework for action *(6)*: sections 5.2 and 6.2).

4.5 Developing capability and capacity
The issue of capacity and workforce development remains a critical issue to be addressed. Responding effectively to implement the social determinants of health and well-being requires action by a broad range of professions and sectors. These would include housing, transport, education, social care, urban planning and design, social protection and environment protection. The shortage of generic skills for the core professions involved in developing and supporting sustainable communities has been identified across the European Region. Action is essential to develop an understanding and appreciation of the social determinants of health and the social gradient and to engage these sectors and professions to meet the demands of the new agenda. The lack of progress often results from lack of awareness of the issues and the contributions of specific professions, agencies and government. This can lead to inertia or obstruction in taking the concerted action necessary (framework for action *(6)*: section 6.2).

4.6 Managing the political environment
The report highlights the importance of securing a place for addressing the social determinants of health on the political agenda and maintaining this to ensure that social policy continues to address the issue in the long term. The core functions of national and local government need to be strengthened, especially in relation to comprehensive understanding of the causes of the causes of inequities in health, participatory governance that engages and empowers individuals and communities and that adopt new roles in creating the conditions in which power is shared and health and well-being are co-produced with citizens and communities. The section on partnership calls for different forms of political and civic leadership focused on participation. It means concerted action by the range of individuals, agencies and all levels of government that can affect the social determinants of health, fostering whole-system approaches to addressing inequities in health (framework for action *(6)*: sections 4.3, 5.4 and 6.1).

4.7 Transferring knowledge
The report has set out the need to further develop systems for transferring knowledge between and within countries in the European Region. This does not mean that initiatives taken in one place will transfer with-

out difficulty elsewhere. The need to address different cultural, historical, political and social contexts is well understood. However, learning networks have been established, and such mechanisms will have added value in the context of global action in relation to the social determinants of health and inequities in health.

References

1. Commission on Social Determinants of Health. *Closing the gap in a generation: health equity through action on the social determinants of health. Final report of the Commission on Social Determinants of Health*. Geneva, World Health Organization, 2008 (http://www.who.int/social_determinants/resources/gkn_lee_al.pdf, accessed 20 April 2012).
2. *Social determinants of health: key concepts*. Geneva, World Health Organization, 2011 (http//:www.who.int/social_determinants/thecommission/finalreport/key_concepts/en/index.html, accessed 20 April 2012).
3. Dalli J. *Pre-inauguration hearings before the European Parliament*. Strasbourg, European Parliament, 2010 (http://www.europarl.europa.eu/hearings/static/commissioners/speeches/dali_speeches_en.pdf, accessed 20 April 2012).
4. *Together for health: a strategic approach for the EU 2008–2013*. Brussels, European Commission, 2007 (http://ec.europa.eu/health/ph_overview/Documents/strategy_wp_en.pdf, accessed 20 April 2012).
5. *Communication from the Commission to the European Parliament, the Council, the European Economic and Social Committee and the Committee of the Regions – solidarity in health: reducing health inequalities in the EU*. Brussels, European Commission, 2009 (http://ec.europa.eu/health/ph_determinants/socio_economics/documents/com2009_en.pdf, accessed 20 April 2012).
6. *Healthy cities tackle the social determinants of inequities in health: a framework for action*. Copenhagen, WHO Regional Office for Europe, 2012.
7. *The European health report 2009: health and health systems*. Copenhagen, WHO Regional Office for Europe, 2009 (http://www.euro.who.int/__data/assets/pdf_file/0009/82386/E93103.pdf, accessed 20 April 2012).
8. Knowledge Network on Urban Settings of the Commission on Social Determinants of Health. *Our cities, our health, our future: acting on social determinants for health equity in urban settings*. Kobe, WHO Centre for Health Development, 2008 (http://www.who.int/entity/social_determinants/resources/knus_final_report_052008.pdf, accessed 20 April 2012).
9. Barton H, Tsourou C. *Healthy urban planning: a WHO guide to planning for people*. London, Spon, 2000.
10. Saltman RB, Bankauskaite V. Central issues in the decentralization debate. In: Saltman RB, Bankauskaite V, Vrangbaek K, eds. *Decentralization in healthcare*. Maidenhead, Open University Press, 2007.
11. Litvack J, Ahmad J, Bird R. *Rethinking decentralization in developing countries*. Washington, DC, World Bank, 1998 (http://siteresources.worldbank.org/INTHSD/Resources/topics/Stewardship/Rethinking_Decentralization.pdf, accessed 20 April 2012).
12. De Vries MS. The rise and fall of decentralization: a comparative analysis of arguments and practices in European countries. *European Journal of Political Research*, 2000, 38:193–224 (http://www.ru.nl/aspx/download.aspx?File=/contents/pages/140660/ejprdecentralization.pdf, accessed 20 April 2012).
13. Mitchell G, Dorling D. An environmental justice analysis of British air quality. *Environment and Planning*, 2003, A35:909–929.

14. Lavin T et al. *Health effects of the built environment*. Dublin, Institute of Public Health, 2006.
15. Whitley R, Prince M. Fear of crime and mental health in inner city London. *Social Science and Medicine*, 2005, 61:1678–1688.
16. Naess Ø et al. Air pollution, social deprivation, and mortality: a multilevel cohort study. *Epidemiology*, 2007, 18:686–694.
17. Forastiere F et al. Socio-economic status, particulate air pollution and daily mortality: differential exposure or differential susceptibility. *American Journal of Industrial Medicine*, 2007, 50:208–216.
18. Grayling T et al. *Streets ahead: safe and liveable streets for children*. London, Institute for Public Policy Research, 2002.
19. Royal Commission on Environmental Pollution. *Twenty-sixth report: the urban environment*. London, The Stationery Office, 2007.
20. Ellaway A, Macintyre S, Bonnefoy X. Graffiti, greenery and obesity in adults: secondary analysis of European cross-sectional survey. *British Medical Journal*, 2005, 331:611–612.
21. Grant M. *Health inequalities and determinants in the physical urban environment*. Bristol, WHO Collaborating Centre for Healthy Cities, University of the West of England, 2010.
22. Mitchell R, Popham F. Effects of the exposure to the natural environment on health inequalities: an observational population study. *Lancet*, 2008, 372:1655–1660.
23. Croucher K et al. *Health and the physical characteristics of urban neighbourhood: a critical literature review. Final report*. Glasgow, Glasgow Centre for Population Health, 2007.
24. Horowitz K, McKay M. Community violence and urban families: experience, effect and direction for intervention. *American Journal of Orthopsychiatry*, 2005, 75:356–368.
25. Buzeti T et al. *Health inequalities in Slovenia*. Ljubljana, National Institute of Public Health, 2011 (http://www.euro.who.int/__data/assets/pdf_file/0008/131759/Health_inequalities_in_Slovenia.pdf, accessed 20 April 2012).
26. *Fair society, healthy lives: strategic review of health inequalities in England post-2010*. London, Marmot Review, 2010.
27. Wilkinson R, Pickett K. *The spirit level: why equality is better for everyone*. London, Penguin Books, 2010.
28. Peake S et al. *Health equity through intersectoral action: an analysis of 18 country case studies*. Ottawa, Public Health Agency of Canada and Geneva, World Health Organization, 2008 (http://www.who.int/pmnch/topics/health_systems/healthequity_who/en/index.html, accessed 20 April 2012).
29. Early Child Development Knowledge Network of the Commission on Social Determinants of Health. *Early child development: a powerful equalizer – final report of the Early Child Development Knowledge Network*. Geneva, World Health Organization, 2007 (http://www.who.int/social_determinants/publications/earlychilddevelopment/en/index.html, accessed 20 April 2012).
30. Conti G, Heckman J, Zanolini A. The developmental origins of health: cognition, personality, and education. *6th Annual Nestle International Nutrition Symposium, Lausanne, Switzerland, 22 October 2009*.
31. Allen G. *Early interventions: the next steps*. London, Cabinet Office, 2011.
32. Cummings C et al. *Evaluation of the Full Service Extended Schools Initiative: final report*. London, Department for Education and Skills, 2007.

33. Stewart-Brown S. *What is the evidence on school health promotion in improving health or preventing disease and, specifically, what is the effectiveness of the health promoting schools approach?* Copenhagen, WHO Regional Office for Europe, 2006 (http://www.euro.who.int/document/e88185.pdf, accessed 20 April 2012).
34. Morris J et al. A minimum income for healthy living. *Journal of Epidemiology and Community Health*, 2000, 54:885–889.
35. *The London health inequalities strategy.* London, Greater London Authority, 2010.
36. Matrix Evidence Ltd. *Valuing health: developing a business case for health improvement.* London, Improvement and Development Agency, 2009.
37. Lyons M. *National prosperity, local choice and civic engagement: a new partnership between central and local government for the 21st century.* London, HMT, 2006.
38. Perkins N et al. *What counts is what works? New Labour and partnership on public health.* Bristol, Policy Press, 2009.
39. *No more toxic assets.* London, Commission for Architecture and the Built Environment, 2009.
40. Boyce T, Patel S. *The health impact of spatial planning decisions.* London, Kings Fund, 2009.
41. Parkes A, Kearns A. *The multi-dimensional neighbourhood and health. A cross sectional analysis of the Scottish Household Survey 2001.* Bristol, ESRC Centre for Neighbourhood Research, 2004 (CNR Paper 19).
42. *Healthy lives, healthy people: our strategy for public health in England.* London, Department of Health, 2010.
43. *Tackling health inequalities: 10 years on.* London, Department of Health, 2009.
44. *Regionalism across Europe.* Brussels, Assembly of European Regions, 2006.
45. *The state of regionalism in Europe: an AER report.* Brussels, Assembly of European Regions, 2010.
46. Strandberg-Larsen M et al. Denmark: health system review. *Health Systems in Transition*, 2007, 9(6):1–164.
47. Tragakes E et al. Latvia: health system review. *Health Systems in Transition*, 2008, 10(2):1–253.
48. *Compendium of cultural policies and trends in Europe.* 12th ed. Strasbourg, Council of Europe, 2011 (http://www.culturalpolicies.net/web/latvia.php?aid=22, accessed 20 April 2012).
49. Vallgarda S. Social inequality in health: dichotomy or gradient? A comparative study of problematizations in national public health programmes. *Health Policy*, 2007, 85:71–82.
50. Judge K et al. *Health inequalities: a challenge for Europe.* London, United Kingdom Presidency of the European Union, 2006 (http://ec.europa.eu/health/ph_determinants/socio_economics/ev_060302_rd05_en.pdf, accessed 20 April 2012).
51. Barton H, Mitcham C, Tsourou C, eds. *Healthy urban planning in practice: experience of European cities.* Copenhagen, WHO Regional Office for Europe, 2003 (http://www.euro.who.int/__data/assets/pdf_file/0003/98400/E82657.pdf, accessed 20 April 2012).
52. Mackenbach JP, Bakker MJ. Tackling socioeconomic inequalities in health: analysis of European experiences. *Lancet*, 2003, 362:1409–1414.
53. Stokke O, Foster J, eds. *Policy coherence in developmental cooperation.* London, Frank Cass, 1999 (EADI Book Series 22).
54. Smithies J, Hampson S. *Review of good practice in community participation and health projects and initiatives.* Howarth, Labyrinth Consultancy and Training, 1999.
55. Andern J. *Social exclusion and inclusion in the globalised city.* Roskilde, Roskilde University, 2004.
56. Cook B. *Health inequalities.* Belfast, Southern Health Board, Northern Ireland, 2009.